Politics and Healthcare

Where is Nursing?

By

Sue Johnson

Politics and Healthcare: Where is Nursing?

By Sue Johnson

This book first published 2024

Ethics International Press Ltd, UK

British Library Cataloguing in Publication Data

A catalogue record for this book is available from the British Library

Print Book ISBN: 978-1-80441-527-6

eBook ISBN: 978-1-80441-528-3

TABLE OF CONTENTS

PREFACE

The true forms of government, therefore, are those in which the one, or the few, or the many, govern with a view to the common interest; but governments which rule with a view to the private interest, whether of the one or of the few, or of the many, are perversions. For the members of a state, if they are truly citizens, ought to participate in its advantages.

—Aristotle

Politics frequently have a negative connotation today. Yet politics are a fact of our daily life. We encounter politics when we read the morning paper, watch a news program, chat on the Internet, and talk with others at work, church, school, civic organizations, volunteer occasions, and even at home. Nurses have numerous opportunities to engage in politics on the local level and often avoid them like the plague.

This book is a different view of politics and the role it plays in our everyday lives. It uses a historic perspective to define politics and its influence on health care and nursing from our nation's founding to today. It explores why nurses must use their knowledge and expertise to engage in the political process for the sake of their patients, community, colleagues, family, and themselves.

Nurses must be informed citizens of our republic. That sounds easy, but there are multiple ramifications for policy issues and staying informed and updated is a challenge. The process begins with awareness and progresses to knowledge and involvement even on a small scale. Nurses understand how the social determinants of health (SDOH) impact the health and safety of their fellow Americans, especially minority, underserved, and rural populations. The voices of nurses are essential for creating policies to address these needs and educate leaders at all levels to support these individuals.

Several nurses who have navigated the political process locally, regionally, and nationally share their stories of success and challenges. Their advice is invaluable for nurses who are unsure about how to begin.

Where do we go from here? Politics is what we make it—positive, negative, or neutral. Nurses have an opportunity to lead the way to healthcare equity and system changes that benefit everyone and that starts locally. The information here is a starting point, not the end of the journey.

INTRODUCTION

All politics is local in the last analysis.

—Price, Thomas P. 1932

This quote was popularized by Speaker of the House Thomas P. "Tip" O'Neill, Jr. in his first political campaign in 1935. It's important for nurses to remember this as they become politically aware. In the greater scheme of things, why does it matter?

Two reasons come to mind:

1. Nurses are the most trusted profession and
2. Nurses are the largest healthcare profession in the United States.

The Gallup Poll has ranked nursing as the most trusted profession annually except for 2001 after the September 11 attacks. For 21 years, nurses are national leaders in ethics and honesty (Advisory Board, 2023 & ana.org, 2023). While this is good news, there is a caveat. The 79% very high or high rating for nurses in 2023 is the lowest percentage since 2014. In comparison, the professions rated least honest and ethical were members of Congress (63%) and telemarketers (59%) (Advisory Board, 2023).

Much of the data for health professions is from 2020–2021. The 2020 National Nursing Workforce Survey revealed that there are almost 4.2 million RNs and 950,000 LPNs or LVNs in the United States. That is 4 times as many nurses than physicians. So in the U.S.: nursing careers make up the largest portion of America's healthcare professions (usa.edu, 2021).

With this information in mind, why does it matter if nurses are politically aware and involved? The obvious response is nurses have the prestige and numbers to advocate for health care changes that will benefit our society.

Why doesn't this occur routinely?

- Is it lack of awareness about issues?
- Is it lack of education in navigating the political process?
- Is it lack of desire to get involved?
- Is it fear of failure?
- Is it lack of confidence in own persuasive skills and abilities?
- Is it the lack of taking a stand that may be unpopular?
- Is it lack of support by friends or colleagues?
- It is lack of time?

There are probably myriad reasons nurses avoid involvement which brings us to the saying at the beginning, "All politics is local in the last analysis" (Price, 1932). Nurses live and work in their own communities. Their children go to local schools. They buy groceries and supplies locally. They participate in local organizations. They have family, friends, and acquaintances locally. They see changes that should be made to improve the community. Their initial response may be to study positions of school board candidates and vote for the best person for the position. From there, they can increase their involvement in political advocacy as their comfort increases.

Think of the power of 4.2 million nurses, members of the most trusted profession, as they truly make a difference in the political canvas of the United States—one step at a time!

—Sue Johnson

1

WHAT IS POLITICS?

Politics is the master science through which individuals collectively set structure, purpose, and ideals in their lives. Politics, therefore, does not emerge from the activities of a single individual but from that of many.

—Aristotle, n.d.

Aristotle's definition of politics is one of many, and scholars do not agree on a uniform definition. Let's examine how politics has different meanings depending on the definition and how these meanings affect its use in practice.

Politics is	Politics includes	This definition excludes
that which concerns the state	permanent institutions that provide public services, ensure security, enforce laws, and regulate the conduct of those in their jurisdictions	the many political activities that don't directly involve the state
a non-violent method of conflict resolution	peaceful negotiation and arbitration to solve problems	the possibility that differences and conflict may be desirable
conflict	respect for those who are different and conflict is organized and productive	conflict resolution as the only desirable outcome
the exercise of power	influence over the actions of others and distribution of resources	a single definition of power–narrow or broad

(*continued*)

Politics is	Politics includes	This definition excludes
a social activity	interactions and dialogue with each other	if everything that is social is or is not political
a public activity	an action directed outward in the public or private sector	attempts to preserve the status quo
dependent on context and interpretation	everything potentially may be political depending on the situation and how it is interpreted	the intention of those performing an action
a struggle over the meaning of political concepts	lack of agreement about terms and criteria	where politics begins and ends

(The Open University, 2019)

As shown in the chart, definitions vary, overlap, and move from a narrower perspective to a broader one. It is essential to critically consider these competing definitions of politics and understand that they are not mutually exclusive.

Another way to define politics is based on scholars' definitions over time. Aristotle's quote is one of many interpretations of the word. He believed that every individual action is political in nature and that politics is essentially the study of ethics and values, right and wrong, and what should be and could be. He believed that communication between two people involves these subjects and is political in nature (Aristotle, n.d.).

Other scholars defined politics differently. Machiavelli, the 16th century philosopher, is widely considered to be the founder of modern political theory. He stated that politics is the study of power, and that political leaders may use any means necessary to strengthen the political institution and preserve authority, peace, and stability. In order to ensure the development of strong and stable societies, he advocated for the separation of church and state (Rose, 2018).

Harold Lasswell was a leading American political scientist in the 20th century. He believed politics were based on who gains and who loses. He focused on power dynamics to determine the distribution of values or desired goals in society. Power was the ability to participate in decision-making, and political power had the ability to produce intended effects on other people. Lasswell considered the opinions and actions of those in power to influence nearly all forms of public policy implemented at all government levels (Rose, 2018).

Jeff Stonecash is currently one of the foremost experts on the American political system, and his definition is a broad one.

Stonecash believes that politics is all-encompassing and includes the study of opportunities, individual responsibilities and beliefs, and the government's role in making these possible (Rose, 2018).

Scholars have also debated whether or not politics is a science like physics, chemistry, or biology. Although it deals with intangible concepts and theoretical assumptions that are difficult to measure and record, it is a form of science because the scientific method is used in every new political theory to test its validity. Political scientists also differ from politicians in several ways.

Political Scientists' Approaches	Politicians' Approaches
Measured, well-thought-out responses to policy questions	Quick answers to policy questions to appeal to voters
Reach tentative conclusions after understanding the facts behind a political issue	Tend to hold firm in their views to appeal to voter base and stay in tune with their ideologies
Seek accuracy and measured responses	Seek ways to expand their popularity and improve chances of reelection

(Rose, 2018)

What is politics? Is it an art, a science, or both? What impact, if any, does it have on our daily life? How would you define it based on the above information? These are questions you must ask yourself as you explore this book. You may find that your current definition of politics changes as you learn more about American politics and the role of nurses in today's political process.

2

THE UNITED STATES—BIRTH OF A REPUBLIC

When in the Course of Human Events, it becomes necessary for one People to dissolve the Political Bands which have connected them with another, and to assume among the Powers of the Earth, the separate and equal Station to which the Laws of Nature and of Nature's God entitle them, a decent Respect to the Opinions of Mankind required that they should declare the causes which impel them to the Separation.

Declaration of Independence, 1776

This quote prefaces the Declaration of Independence of the United States and is an excellent beginning to any study of politics in the United States. In the summer of 1776, colonial representatives in Philadelphia were interested in justifying their decision to declare independence from Great Britain. As Jefferson, Adams, Franklin, and the others realized, this document had to do more than discredit British rule. It became the template for the future American government—one that still exists today. Jefferson's statement that "We hold these truths to be self-evident" invokes the belief that human law is derived from a natural law of right and wrong. Everyone is capable of moral reasoning that enables them to question laws and change them if needed; this is the foundation of today's political system (Cato Institute, 2013).

The Declaration of Independence delineates colonists' grievances against King George III and his government. The representatives of the Thirteen Colonies took a radical step that created the United States of America by dissolving all allegiance to Great Britain and declaring the colonies "Free and Independent States." The Declaration further outlines the power of the new United States "to levy war, conclude peace, contract alliances, establish commerce, and do all other acts and things which independent states may of right do."

In 1787, another meeting occurred in Philadelphia to draft a plan to govern the new nation. Some of the original participants were there along with others sent to represent their respective states. At the Constitutional Convention James Madison of Virginia became a leading force in developing the document with input from other delegates. Their work was based on the Declaration of Independence and designed to create a government strong enough to prevent domestic and foreign oppression with a system of checks and balances. The United States had fought a long war to achieve liberty from government oppression and they were not about to endow their new government with absolute power. As the Preamble states,

> We the People of the United States, in Order to form a more perfect Union, establish Justice, insure domestic Tranquility, provide for the common defence, promote the general Welfare, and secure the Blessings of Liberty to ourselves and our Posterity, do ordain and establish this Constitution for the United States of America.

Power belonged to the people, but they delegated limited and specific powers to the government to exercise on their behalf; this was intentional. The Constitution created three branches of the federal government: legislative, executive, and judicial.

The legislative branch is defined in Article I, which outlines the membership and duties of the Senate and House of Representatives. The House of Representatives has the power to impeach and originate all bills for raising revenue, while the Senate has the power to try all impeachments and propose or concur with amendments to such bills. Congress' powers include:

> "To lay and collect Taxes, Duties. Imposts and Excises;
>
> "To pay the Debts and provide for the common Defense and general Welfare of the United States;
>
> "To borrow Money on the credit of the United States;

"To regulate Commerce with foreign Nations and among the several States, and with the Indian tribes;

"To establish a uniform Rule of Naturalization, and uniform Laws on the subject of Bankruptcies throughout the United States;

"To coin Money, regulate the Value thereof, and of foreign Coin, and fix the Standard of Weights and Measures;

"To provide for the Punishment of counterfeiting the Securities and current Coin of the United States;

"To establish Post Offices and post Roads;

"To promote the Progress of Science and useful Arts, by securing for limited Times to Authors and Inventors the exclusive Right to their respective Writings and Discoveries;

"To constitute Tribunals inferior to the supreme Court;

"To define and punish Piracies and Felonies committed on the high Seas, and Offenses against the law of Nations;

"To declare War, grant Letters of Marque and Reprisal, and make rules concerning Captures on Land and Water;

"To raise and support Armies, but no Appropriation of Money to that Use shall be for a longer Term than two Years;

"To provide and maintain a Navy;

"To make Rules for the Government and Regulation of the land and naval Forces;

"To provide for calling forth the Militia to execute the Laws of the Union, suppress Insurrections and repel Invasions;

"To provide for organizing, arming, and disciplining, the Militia, and for governing such Part of them as may be employed in the Service of the United States;

> "To exercise exclusive Legislation over such District (not exceeding ten Miles square) as may become the Seat of the Government of the United States; and
>
> "To make all Laws which shall be necessary and proper for carrying into Execution the foregoing Powers, and all other Powers vested by this Constitution in the Government of the United States, or in any Department or Officer thereof" (U.S. Const. art. I, § 8).

The states retained legislative authority in appointing officers and training militia. The delegates also ensured that:

> "The Privilege of the Writ of Habeas Corpus shall not be suspended, unless when in Cases of Rebellion or Invasion the Public Safety may require it;
>
> "No bill of attainder or ex post facto Law shall be passed;
>
> "No Capitation, or other direct, Tax shall be laid, unless in Proportion to the Census or Enumeration herein before directed to be taken (requirement removed in the Sixteenth Amendment);
>
> "No Tax or Duty shall be laid on Articles exported from any State;
>
> "No Preference shall be given by any Regulation of Commerce or Revenue to the Ports of one State over those of another;
>
> "No Money shall be drawn from the Treasury, but in Consequence of Appropriations made by Law; and a regular Statement and Account of the Receipts and Expenditures of all public Money shall be published from time to time; and
>
> "No Title of Nobility shall be granted by the United States; And no Person holding any Office of Profit or Trust under them, shall, without the Consent of the Congress, accept of any present, Emolument, Office, or Title, of any kind whatever, from any King, Prince, or foreign State" (U.S. Const. art. I, § 9).

The Constitution also constrained States from the following:

> "No State shall enter into any Treaty, Alliance, or Confederation;
>
> "grant Letters of Marque and Reprisal;
>
> "coin Money;
>
> "emit Bills of Credit;
>
> "make any Thing but gold and silver Coin a Tender in Payment of Debts;
>
> "pass any Bill of Attainder, ex post facto Law, or Law impairing the Obligation of Contracts or;
>
> "grant any Title of Nobility" (U.S. Const. art. I, § 10).

Consent by Congress was needed for States to:

> "lay any Imposts or Duties on Imports or Exports, except what may be absolutely necessary for executing its inspection Laws: and the net Produce of all Duties and Imposts, laid by any State on Imports or Exports, shall be for the Use of the Treasury of the United States; and
>
> "lay the Duty of Tonnage, keep Troops, or Ships of War in time of Peace, enter into any Agreement or Compact with another State, or with a foreign Power, or engage in War, unless actually invaded, or in such imminent Danger as will not admit of delay" (U.S. Const. art. I, § 10).

Although the language is antiquated, the intent of this section of the Constitution is clear—to define the roles and responsibilities of Congress and the respective States.

Article II defines the executive branch, including the requirements and duties of the president, vice president, and civil officers. When the Constitution was written, the most common form of government internationally was the monarchy, and the delegates had not escaped one monarchy to create another. Aristotle described monarchy in two forms: a perpetual, hereditary generalship, and absolute royalty. He maintained that there are three forms of government—royalty, aristocracy, and constitutional. In his own words,

> . . . where men are alike and equal, it is neither expedient nor just that one man should be lord of all, whether there are laws, or whether there are no laws, but he himself is in the place of law.
>
> —Aristotle, n.d.

His views on constitutional government also influenced the delegates at the Constitutional Convention:

> . . . the people who are suited for constitutional freedom are those among whom there naturally exists a warlike multitude able to rule and to obey in turn by a law which gives office to the well-to-do according to their desert.
>
> —Aristotle, n.d.

Article II describes the term of office for the president and vice president and implements the Electoral College, which still exists today. Since there were no political parties at that time, the electors, who could not include any senator or representative, "shall meet in their respective States, and vote by Ballot for two Persons, of whom one at least shall not be an Inhabitant of the same State with themselves" (U.S. Const. art. II, § 1). The list of votes was submitted to the president of the Senate who opened all ballots in the presence of both the Senate and House of Representatives. The top vote-getter became president, and the person receiving the next number of votes became vice president.

The president was required to take an oath when entering office that continues today: "I do solemnly swear (or affirm) that I will faithfully execute the Office of President of the United States, and will to the best of my Ability, preserve, protect and defend the Constitution of the United States" (U.S. Const. art. II, § 1). The president received certain powers during their term in office. These powers included:

> "...shall be Commander in Chief of the Army and Navy of the United States, and of the Militia of the several States, when called into the actual Service of the United States;

> "...may require the Opinion, in writing, of the principal Officer in each of the executive Departments, upon any Subject relating to the Duties of their respective Offices;
>
> "...grant Reprieves and Pardons for Offenses against the United States, except in Cases of Impeachment;
>
> "...fill up all Vacancies that may happen during the Recess of the Senate, by granting Commissions which shall expire at the End of their next Session;
>
> "...receive Ambassadors and other public Ministers;
>
> "...take Care that the Laws be faithfully executed; and
>
> "shall Commission all the Officers of the United States" (U.S. Const. art. II).

A system of checks and balances was designed to prevent the president from executing absolute power; this included Advice and Consent of the Senate:

> "to make treaties, provided two thirds of the Senators present concur; and
>
> nominate, and by and with the Advice and Consent of the Senate, shall appoint Ambassadors, other public Ministers and Consuls, Judges of the supreme Court and all other Officers of the United States, whose Appointments are not herein otherwise provided for, and which shall be established by Law" (U.S. Const. art. II, § 2).

Congress also had the right to "vest the appointment of such inferior officers, as they think proper, in the President alone...or in the Heads of Departments" (U.S. Const. art. II, § 2). The President was also required periodically to report to Congress on the State of the Union and recommend "to their Consideration such Measures as he shall judge necessary and expedient" (U.S. Const. art. II, § 3). Even the President's power to veto legislation was subject to override by two-thirds of the House of Representatives and Senate (U.S. Const. art. I, § 7).

Article III addresses judicial power. According to this section, "The judicial Power of the United States, shall be vested in one supreme Court, and in such inferior Courts as the Congress may from time to time ordain and establish" (U.S. Const. art. III, § 1). Rather than specific terms of office such as Congress and the president, judges appointed to all courts "shall hold their Offices during good Behavior" and their power extended to:

> "all Cases, in Law and Equity, arising under this Constitution, the Laws of the United States, and Treaties made, or which shall be made, under their Authority;
>
> "all Cases affecting Ambassadors, other public Ministers and Consuls;
>
> "all Cases of admiralty and maritime Jurisdiction;
>
> "Controversaries to which the United States shall be a Party; and
>
> "Controversaries between two or more States; between Citizens of different States; between Citizens of the same State claiming Lands under Grants under different States [and between a State, or the Citizens thereof, and foreign States, Citizens or Subjects]" (U.S. Const. art. III, § 2). This was subsequently changed by the Eleventh Amendment: "The Judicial power of the United States shall not be construed to extend to any suit in law or equity, commenced or prosecuted against one of the United States by Citizens of another State, or by Citizens or Subjects of any Foreign State" (U.S. Const. amend. XI).

Article III also delineates trial by jury except in cases of impeachment and defines treason against the United States with Congress determining punishment.

Article IV deals with state and citizen rights and Article V addresses the process for proposing amendments to the Constitution. Proposed amendments must be ratified by the legislatures of three fourths on the states, ensuring that the federal government doesn't overreach its power in the governing process. The Constitution became "the supreme Law of the Land" and all leaders in Congress, in state legislatures, and all executive and judicial officers are required "by Oath or Affirmation, to support this Constitution" (U.S. Const. art. VI).

The Constitution remains a living document to ensure that powers not granted to the three branches of government will reside in the people of the United States. A system of checks and balances is designed to guarantee that liberty endures. It remains unique and valid today in our Republic and in the world.

3

THE AMERICAN REPUBLIC

That all things should be decided by all is characteristic of democracy; this is the sort of equality which the people desire.

—Aristotle, n.d.

Many people believe the United States is a democracy because the framers of the Constitution stated, "The United States shall guarantee to every State in this Union a Republican Form of Government" (U.S. Const. art. IV, § 4). This led to a conversation between Elizabeth Powel, the wife of Philadelphia Mayor Samuel Powel, and Benjamin Franklin, which was recorded by Dr. James McHenry, a Maryland delegate. Although he edited the conversation years later, the original quote in 1787 was:

"Powel: Well Doctor, what have we got—a republic or a monarchy?"

"Franklin: A republic, if you can keep it" (Bell, 2017).

The words democracy and republic are not interchangeable, and their functions are different. Perhaps the best description of the two was from James Madison in *The Federalist Papers* on November 23, 1787. Madison was a proponent of republican government. In Federalist No. 10 he expressed concern about dangers to the new government and how to address them. The Constitution has not totally prevented these dangers, particularly those of factions or groups united by common interests that are "adverse to the rights of other citizens, or to the permanent and aggregate interests of the community" (Madison, 1787). These groups could be either a majority or minority, but their influence could taint public administrations and create "distrust of public engagements, and alarm for private rights" (Madison, 1787).

Madison believed that such factions or groups must be dealt with and recommended "two methods of curing the mischiefs of faction: the one, by removing its causes; the other, by controlling its effects" (Madison, 1787). According to Madison, it is not practical to remove the causes by destroying liberty or making every citizen have the same interests, opinions, and passions. Liberty is essential to political life and there will always be different interests, opinions, and passions. Therefore, it would be impossible to remove the causes of these factions or groups. The only alternative is to control their effects. Minority factions can be controlled by regular voting. When a majority faction is present, it is essential to "secure the public good and the rights of other citizens, and at the same time to preserve the spirit and the form of popular government" (Madison, 1787), leading to Madison's definitions of a democracy and a republic.

As illustrated in the table (see below), Madison lent his support to the Republic, believing that its advantages outweighed its weakness. The Constitution was designed to address the Republic's weakness with "the great and aggregate interests being referred to the national, the local and particular to the State legislatures" (Madison, 1787). Representatives selected by more citizens were more likely to keep the Union secure by preventing one party from outnumbering and oppressing the rest.

When the Constitution was ratified in 1789 as a Republic, the Union was difficult to establish. The country was large with sectional differences, arduous travel, and slow, unreliable communication. Americans put the interest of their state or region ahead of the country and many opposed the Constitution as threatening states' rights and individual liberty. The Constitution, as previously discussed, did not alleviate these concerns. John Adams of Massachusetts was concerned that there was no bill of rights like the one he had written for the Massachusetts Constitution in 1780 (Handlin, 1966; McCullough, 2001).

In 1789, Adams was the first vice president under George Washington and presided over the Senate. Madison, who had opposed a bill of rights earlier, now became its most vocal proponent. When Massachusetts balked at ratifying the Constitution, adding rights-related amendments became imperative (archives.gov). Because citizens within the states were concerned about potential abuse of power by the federal government, the Senate and House of Representatives met in New York City to consider adding rights-related amendments that would make

Democracy	Republic
Definition: "a society consisting of a small number of citizens, who assemble and administer the government in person"	**Definition:** "a government in which the scheme of representation takes place"
Delegation of the government: "A small number of citizens elected by the rest"	**Delegation of the government:** "Greater number of citizens and greater sphere of country, over which the latter may be extended"
Philosophy: "by reducing mankind to a perfect equality in their political rights, they would, at the same time, be perfectly equalized and assimilated in their possessions, their opinions, and their passions"	**Philosophy**: "To secure the public good and private rights, and at the same time to preserve the spirit and form of popular government"
Sphere of Control: Narrow	**Sphere of Control:** Broad
Advantage: Confined to a small region "The smaller the society, the fewer probably will be the distinct parties and interests composing it; the fewer the distinct parties and interests, the more frequently will a majority be found of the same party."	**Advantage:** Extended over a large region "Extend the sphere, and you take in a greater variety of parties and interests; you make it less probably that a majority of the whole will have a common motive to invade the rights of other citizens; or if such a common motive exists, it will be more difficult for all who feel it to discover their own strength, and to act in unison with each other."
Weaknesses: "there is nothing to check the inducements to sacrifice the weaker party or an obnoxious individual;" "incompatible with personal security or the rights of property"	**Weaknesses:** "By enlarging too much the number of electors, you render the representatives too little acquainted with all their local circumstances and lesser interests; as by reducing it too much, you render him unduly attached to these and too little fit to comprehend and pursue great and national projects"

(Madison, 1787)

the Constitution more palatable to the states. In June 1787, Madison introduced a list of amendments designed to reflect the importance of these protections to citizens. He also believed that including them in the Constitution would educate people about their rights and prevent more drastic changes to the document. The House subsequently passed a joint resolution with 17 amendments based on Madison's list. The Senate reduced the number of amendments to 12 and a joint Senate and House Conference Committee agreed on the 12 amendments (archives.gov).

Then, copies of the 12 amendments were sent to each state in October 1789 for ratification. For reasons previously mentioned, this was a lengthy process. However, by December 1791, three-fourths of the 13 state legislatures ratified 10 of these amendments. The other 2 that concerned Congressional representation and Congressional pay were not adopted at that time (Cato Institute, 2013).

The first 10 Amendments to the Constitution are commonly called the Bill of Rights and include:

> **Amendment I**—"Congress shall make no law respecting an establishment of religion, or prohibiting the free exercise thereof; or abridging the freedom of speech, or of the press, or the right of the people peaceably to assemble, and to petition the Government for a redress of grievances";
>
> **Amendment II**—"A well-regulated Militia, being necessary to the security of a free State, the right of the people to keep and bear Arms, shall not be infringed";
>
> **Amendment III**—"No Soldier shall, in time of peace be quartered in any house, without the consent of the Owner, nor in time of war, but in a manner to be prescribed by law";
>
> **Amendment IV**—"The right of the people to be securer in their persons, houses, papers, and effects, against unreasonable searches and seizures, shall not be violated, and no Warrants shall issue, but upon probable cause, supported by Oath or affirmation, and particularly describing the place to be searched, and the persons or things to be seized";
>
> **Amendment V**—"No person shall be held to answer for a capital, or otherwise infamous crime, unless on a presentation or indictment of a Grand Jury, except in cases arising in the land or naval forces, or in the Militia, when in actual service in time of War or public danger; nor shall any person be subject for the same offense to be twice put in jeopardy of life or limb, nor shall be compelled in any criminal case to be a witness

against himself, nor be deprived of life, liberty, or property, without due process of law; nor shall private property be taken for public use without just compensation";

Amendment VI—"In all criminal prosecutions, the accused shall enjoy the right to a speedy and public trial, by an impartial jury of the State and district wherein the crime shall have been committed; which district shall have been previously ascertained by law, and to be informed of the nature and cause of the accusation; to be confronted with the witnesses against him; to have compulsory process for obtaining witnesses in his favor, and to have the assistance of counsel for his defense";

Amendment VII—"In Suits at common law, where the value in controversy shall exceed twenty dollars, the right of trial by jury shall be preserved, and no fact tried by a jury shall be otherwise re-examined in any Court of the United States, than according to the rules of the common law";

Amendment VIII—"Excessive bail shall not be required, nor excessive fines imposed, nor cruel and unusual punishments inflicted";

Amendment IX—"The enumeration in the Constitution of certain rights shall not be construed to deny or disparage other retained by the people"; and

Amendment X—"The powers not delegated to the United States by the Constitution, nor prohibited by it to the States, are reserved to the States respectively, or to the people" (Cato Institute, 2013).

The Bill of Rights is profoundly important to all United States citizens. A bill of rights existed in several states during the time the Constitution was written and delegates didn't see the need to include one in that document. However, when Massachusetts was reluctant to ratify the Constitution, threatening its existence, circumstances changed. Madison originally opposed adding amendments to the Constitution, believing that they would adversely impact the limited government defined in the Constitution. As he reached the conclusion that these rights could be framed to prevent the abuse of powers not explicitly granted to the government, he first recommended that they be included within the Constitution. The members of the First Congress did not agree with his recommendation, but he led writing proposed amendments to be sent to each state for ratification anyway (Postell, 2007).

Only 10 of the 12 amendments were subsequently ratified, and they were not called the Bill of Rights. Each amendment was voted on separately and reflected rights defined in the Declaration of Independence: "...all Men are created equal, that they are endowed by their Creator with certain unalienable Rights, that among these are Life, Liberty, and the Pursuit of Happiness—That to secure these Rights, Governments are instituted among Men, deriving their just Powers from the consent of the Governed..." (Declaration of Independence, 1776).

These amendments did not attempt to identify all citizen rights and privileges. They also do not say how to safeguard "individual liberty from tyranny of the majority" (Postell, 2007). Madison and his colleagues believed that people must be responsible for the defense of their liberties. These amendments would increase public understanding of their rights and better prepare them to defend these liberties. The first 10 Amendments to the Constitution historically have been called the Bill of Rights, although the term is not found in the document. They did not enlarge the power of the federal government and the 9th and 10th Amendments served as a check on unlimited government. Each individual is unique, and the Bill of Rights serves to safeguard the liberties and privileges of all citizens (Postell, 2007).

The American Republic has endured for nearly 250 years, and these founding documents continue to guide our path as a country today.

4

THE AMERICAN POLITICAL SYSTEM

However [political parties] may now and then answer popular ends, they are likely in the course of time and things, to become potent engines, by which cunning, ambitious, and unprincipled men will be enabled to subvert the power of the people. . .

Washington's Farewell Address on September 19, 1796

As the quote implies, George Washington was opposed to political parties. However, political parties have played a huge role since the beginning of the United States. Washington attempted to circumvent political parties during his administration by appointing two political adversaries to his cabinet in the hopes that they would work together in the national interest. The young nation was threatened by an economic crisis and Washington's appointees—Alexander Hamilton (treasury secretary) and Thomas Jefferson (secretary of state)—had divergent views about how to resolve this crisis (University of Minnesota, 2016).

Hamilton planned to have the federal government assume the debts incurred by the states during the Revolutionary War. His measures included a controversial whiskey tax and the establishment of a national bank. Jefferson and local farmers opposed Hamilton's plan for a whiskey tax, resulting in the Whiskey Rebellion of 1794. Hamilton's response was to bring together a group of powerful supporters to endorse his plan. This group became the Federalist Party, initially at the federal level. The Federalists soon spread to states, counties, and towns, particularly in the Northeast. Hamilton used his military and business connections to develop the Federalist Party at the grassroots level (University of Minnesota, 2016).

Since voting rights had increased during the Revolutionary War, the Federalists wanted to attract voters to their cause using the new organization to create propaganda and campaign for their candidates. They created several newspapers in large cities and smaller ones in rural locations. This partisan press began some of the key tasks of political parties by influencing public opinion and expressing positions on issues. Jefferson and Madison began an anti-Federalist movement, which became the foundation for the Republican Party (not today's Republican Party). The Republicans used other newspapers to communicate their views and actions while inspiring local leaders and groups to align themselves with their party. The political parties feared by Washington had come to life (University of Minnesota, 2016).

The Whiskey Rebellion in 1794 ignited fears that the government could be overthrown by violent factions (parties). In 1796, the two political parties became evident in the presidential election. John Adams, a Federalist, barely won over Thomas Jefferson, a Republican. In 1800, the Federalist and Republican members of Congress met formally to nominate the presidential candidates. This practice was a precursor to today's nominating conventions. Upon election, President Thomas Jefferson established a tradition in the United States of political parties as grassroots organizations where small groups joined to represent various interests, select slates of candidates for office, and present platforms on issues (University of Minnesota, 2016).

These two early political parties were largely comprised of political office holders. The Federalists never expanded beyond the wealthy classes, and their influence decreased over the next several years until the election of 1816. The Federalists received few votes in the 1816 election and soon ceased to exist as a party. By 1820, the Republican Party was the only surviving national party. However, the Republicans experienced infighting and developed into two warring factions. These became the National Republicans and Democratic-Republicans (University of Minnesota, 2016).

By 1828, a true two-party system had developed. The Democratic-Republican Party became the Democratic Party, and a branch of the National Republicans became the Whig Party. Andrew Jackson became president with support of the Democratic Party. The period from 1834 until the start of the Civil War was a time of party politics. Both parties used grassroots campaigning to their advantage. There was door-to-door canvassing for voters, picnics, and rallies sponsored by both parties. Voting by citizens was as high as 96% in some states and campaign buttons came into existence. The Whig Party was replaced in 1854 with the Republican Party when the Whigs suffered internal conflicts over patronage and slavery. This new party consisted of former Whigs, unhappy Democrats, and members of a small anti-slavery party—the Free-Soil Party. The Republicans gained influence with the election of Abraham Lincoln as the 16th president in 1861. In the 1860s, cartoonist Thomas Nast created two symbols for the Democrats (donkey) and Republicans (elephant), which still persist today (University of Minnesota, 2016).

Political parties exerted massive power during the post-Civil War era to the Great Depression. Immigrants from Europe settled mainly in urban areas during this time and machine politics was born. Party machines in these cities were run by bosses who demanded loyalty and service in exchange for jobs and support in becoming citizens. These new citizens then voted as the party bosses demanded. Party machines controlled the government in major cities like Boston, New York, and Chicago and used their power to create public improvement projects that employed many of their voters. The system was corrupt, and bosses used their powerful positions to become wealthy. By ensuring employment in exchange for votes, party bosses could elect officials who let the graft continue. Thomas Nast used political cartoons to alert people of the crimes occurring due to party machines, resulting in the ousting and eventual jailing of Boss Tweed in New York City (University of Minnesota, 2016).

While party bosses got rich and some people got work, political machines didn't benefit everyone. As the United States became more industrialized and large corporations formed, greater disparities in wealth became evident. Factories and coal mines presented dangerous working conditions, and farmers faced declining prices for their crops. Reformers blamed corruption and incompetence of party machines for these conditions. They believed that funds for improving social conditions were being diverted into the bosses' pockets while keeping incompetent associates in power. These reformers, called the mugwumps, joined together in the 1880s to form the Progressive Movement. They began reforms to reduce the parties' grip on the electoral system. By 1896, Progressives succeeded in implementing secret ballots in most states. Before people could only vote for one party; now, they could split their ticket and vote for a person from another party. In 2022, straight ticket voting is only offered in six states: Alabama, Indiana (except for at-large races only), Kentucky, Michigan, Oklahoma, and South Carolina (ncsl, 2022). Progressives also advocated for primary elections where the people could participate rather than caucuses where candidates were chosen by party elites. Primaries began in a few states, but it wasn't until the 1970s that they became commonplace (University of Minnesota, 2016).

Progressives instituted a merit system in 1833 for employment in government by passing the Pendleton Act and establishing the civil service. This helped reduce the influence of political machines but did not eliminate them. Progressive reformers were unsuccessful in running for president, and the Great Depression led to new national leadership. Beginning in 1933, President Franklin Delano Roosevelt's New Deal to end the Great Depression also had massive impact on political parties. The government became a pivotal force in ensuring citizens' economic welfare, and Washington, DC became the power center while the power of the president expanded. Political parties became centered in Washington and national party leaders became detached from their local organizations and voters. They also lost the ability to control the policy agenda (University of Minnesota, 2016).

After World War II, presidential candidates pushed their own agendas on issues and independence as they ran for office. Running on a party label, presidents were elected based on personal, not partisan, appeals to the electorate. Political parties began reforms in the late 1960s to show they were responsive to the public. The Democrats acted first to revamp nominating convention delegates to include more average voters. Many state Democratic parties shifted from caucuses, where delegates were selected by party leaders, to primaries where voters had a voice. Republicans followed with reforms that resulted in states adopting primaries. The resulting candidate-centered politics exists today, and candidates develop their own personal campaign organizations and appeal directly to the public through television and social media. Campaign professionals and media consultants develop election strategies and get voters to the polls (University of Minnesota, 2016).

Here is the story of United States political parties:

Dates	Parties	Overview
1789	No formal Party	Washington did not approve of political parties and none were identified during his term of office.
1794–1796	No formal Party	Two factions were forming: Federalists who believed that the central government and wealthy, well-educated classes should hold the most power. Anti-Federalists who believed that the vast majority of ordinary, less educated people had skills and common sense to run the government.

Dates	Parties	Overview
1797	Federalist & Anti-Federalist Party	Federalist party elects John Adams as second President of the U.S. and the *Federalist Papers* explain the Constitution to the American people.
1798	Republican Party	Anti-Federalist party renamed to reflect Republicanism in supporting states' rights and strict interpretation of the Constitution.
1800	Democratic-Republican Party	What was a derogatory term for the new Republican party became accepted by Jeffersonian Republicans.
1815–1816	Federalist Party Democratic-Republican Party	Federalists opposed the War of 1812 and were discredited resulting in massive loss in the 1816 election and leading to the dissolution of the party.
1817–1823	Democratic-Republican Party	Having only one political party resulted in more stable government.
1824	National Republican Party	Two factions of the Democratic-Republican party unified to enhance national defense and develop U.S. resources.
1825–1828	Democratic-Republican Party	The party split into two factions: northern-dominated Republicans and southern-dominated Democrats.
1829	Democrat Party	Jacksonian Democrats removed "Republican" to form the Democrat party.
1834	Whig Party	This was a new name for National Republicans to support reform.
1837–1853	Democrat Party Whig Party	The presidency veered between both parties until 1853 when intra-party divisions destroyed the Whig party.
1854–1869	Republican Party	This party was organized to oppose extension of slavery.
1869–present	Two Party System	The Democrats and Republicans comprise the two major political parties in the United States.

(Adapted from Lachin, 2015: University of Minnesota, 2016)

As the table above shows, we still have a two-party system and although not all-powerful, the Democrat and Republican parties far outnumber Independents in United States elections.

5

INTERSECTION OF POLITICS AND HEALTHCARE

At the start of the war the tale of the medical department was a sorry one. There was practically no organization nor discipline. Surgical instruments were few. Drugs were few and bad; opium and quinine were scarce and ether was then unknown. Trained nurses and scientific nursing did not exist. Blundering assistants called 'mates' were the only help the surgeons had.

—unknown colonial writer cited in Donahue, 2010

Health care during the American Revolution was poor and disorganized as stated by the colonial writer. The majority of nurses in military hospitals established in private homes were men, but a few women were employed to care for soldiers. A resolution by Congress on July 17, 1775, assigned one nurse to every ten patients in these hospitals. This resolution defined the first nurse-patient ratio in the country. General Washington in 1777 ordered that women should be employed as nurses. However, these women mostly cooked and served meals. Some women followed their husbands into battle and cared for them there. Medicine continued to grow and flourish after the Revolution, but it was a male bastion. Women were effectively excluded from healthcare practice (Donahue, 2010).

This situation persisted until the outbreak of the Civil War in 1861. After Lincoln initially requested mobilization of soldiers, Elizabeth Blackwell, the first female American physician, developed the Women's Central Association for Relief in New York City. This organization persuaded a minister and four physicians to go to Washington and seek the establishment of a sanitary commission to advise the army's medical department and investigate the soldiers' health conditions. The proposed commission faced opposition from the military and some members of the government. When this opposition was resolved, President Lincoln established the United States Sanitary Commission in June 1861 to care for the soldiers (Donahue, 2010).

This was the first intersection between politics and health care since the Revolution. The Women's Central Association for Relief served as a branch of the Sanitary Commission. Its role was to coordinate all relief organizations in the country and send nurses to areas with the most need for assistance. Nurses' training was minimal with 1 month of observation and 1 month of hospital work experience. There was a Western and Eastern Sanitary Commission, but they collaborated with each other. The goal of the Sanitary Commission was to ensure soldiers' health in camps, hospitals, and transports. Their first inspection found poor sanitation, hygiene, rations, and lack of space. Physicians were incompetent or poorly qualified and soldiers suffered as a result. Camps were dirty and without medicines or adequate food. The Government Medical Bureau was suspicious when the Sanitary Commission offered supplies and support. However, the situation was dire, and they had to accept the Commission's contributions. The Sanitary Commission distributed supplies and fresh vegetables, improved sanitation, cared for the wounded, and provided significant health work for the army (Donahue, 2010).

Also in June 1861, Simon Cameron, Secretary of War, appointed Dorothea Dix as Superintendent of the Female Nurses of the Union Army. Miss Dix was not a nurse, but a mental health crusader. She was chosen for her organizational skills and charged with organizing hospitals for care delivery, appointing nurses, and directing donated supplies for distribution to the soldiers. She established strict requirements for nurses and the nurse-patient-ratio remained at 1:10. Women who were unable to meet her requirements continued to serve as nurses without compensation or recognition. Her position was abolished at the end of the War and Miss Dix returned to civilian life (Donahue, 2010).

One of the nurses employed by the Sanitary Commission, Mary A. Livermore, later became a leader in the women's suffrage movement and advocated for more education for women. Another Civil War nurse, Clara Barton, also served in 1870 with the International Red Cross in France. On her return home, she sought to create an American Red Cross and finally succeeded in 1882 when the U.S. government ratified the Geneva Convention and officially recognized the Red Cross.

In 1868 the president of the American Medical Association (AMA) recommended education and training for nurses. Women who had influenced the Sanitary Commission during the war founded the New York State Charities Aid Association in 1872 to seek reforms in the care of the sick, paupers, and orphans. They investigated nursing care at Bellevue Hospital and reported their shocking findings. This report resulted in a resolution to the Commissioners of Charity recommending the establishment of a training school for nurses at Bellevue. The commissioners referred the proposal to the medical board and, after overcoming opposition, the commissioners reluctantly designated six wards at Bellevue for nurse training. Training schools subsequently developed in major cities and students were used as a source of free labor for the hospitals (Donahue, 2010).

Health care and nursing slowly continued to evolve in the later part of the nineteenth century, and politics and health care continued to intersect as the United States entered the Spanish-American War in 1898. Congress authorized employing female nurses on a contract basis with salary, lodging, and meals. It did not include medical care for nurses. Conditions were unsanitary and typhoid and yellow fever were rampant. During experiments to determine if yellow fever was a mosquito-borne disease, a nurse named Clara Maass volunteered to be bitten and died as a result. She was the only woman and American to die during the experiment, and in 1976 she became the first American nurse honored with a commemorative U.S. stamp (Donahue, 2010).

The twentieth century created a movement for social reform in the United States. The first White House Conference on Child Welfare occurred in 1910, and in 1912 Congress established the Children's Bureau within the Department of Labor. The Bureau studied infant mortality, rural health care for mothers and infants, and hygiene instruction to promote the life and welfare of children. The agency's efforts resulted in the Sheppard-Towner Act of 1921, which provided grants to states that set up welfare and hygiene services for mothers and children. Nurses began to make home visits and offer health education and screening while funding established child health centers in 45 states and Hawaii. The infant death rate decreased, and the Act became the first federally funded U.S. social welfare program. In 1929 conservative forces in Congress and the AMA combined successfully to oppose the renewal of the Act on the grounds that it was "...unsound in policy, wasteful and extravagant, unproductive of results and tending to promote communism..." (American Medical Association, 1930). Many pediatricians disagreed with this opposition and left the AMA at this time to form the American Academy of Pediatrics (Johnson Lewis, 2019).

When the act was discontinued, many states continued to provide funding in decreased amounts. In the early twentieth century the intersection between politics and health care occurred on a local and national level. Visiting and public health nursing became a force in health care during these years. One nurse spearheaded this movement by establishing a nursing settlement within a New York neighborhood called the Henry Street Settlement. Her name was Lillian Wald, and the year was 1891. When she and another nurse named Mary Brewster decided to live on the Lower East Side and provide nursing care to tenement residents there, she knew she needed financial support. Miss Wald spoke with a philanthropist, Mrs. Solomon (Betty) Loeb, who convinced her son-in-law, Jacob Schiff, to finance the project (Williams, 1948). Once established in the neighborhood, Miss Wald met with the president of the Board of Health and received official approval for her and Mary Brewster to become visiting nurses, completed with official-looking badges. When Mary Brewster retired in 1893, more space was needed to serve the community. Lillian Wald moved to 265 Henry Street with a number of nurses and volunteers. Over the next 40 years, she changed the face of health care in New York City by interacting with local agencies to improve the lives of children who often worked at an early age and didn't attend school or have recreational opportunities. Lillian Wald wouldn't take "no" for an answer, and her research succeeded. She convinced the Board of Health to hire school nurses and pay them from public funds. She also collaborated with a teacher at a nearby school to develop special education classes for children with physical or mental disabilities. Today, these education practices are accepted throughout the United States, but at the time, they were radical ideas. Miss Wald also created the first public playground on Henry Street where children could play. Coaches and volunteers used rooms at Henry Street where children could study and learn using a donated library. She invited visitors to join the staff, and invited volunteers for meals where she lobbied for child labor changes and reform with philanthropists and legislators. Lillian Wald joined commissions to reform tenements, factories, and develop a children's bureau, which was created by the federal government in 1912 (Block, 1969).

This nurse understood the importance of professional and personal contacts to change the culture on the Lower East Side and used her knowledge and research to improve people's lives locally and nationally.

She joined the Social Reform Club where she interacted with influential people in politics, education, and literature. She studied trade unions and became a founding member of the National Women's Trade Union. She served on multiple boards. Her ultimate focus was not political. It was to help individuals lead a better, healthier life. Lillian Wald became a nursing advocate whose work at Henry Street Settlement positively impacted individuals locally, regionally, and nationally (Block, 1969).

Politics and health care continued to intersect in the United States and other nurses used this junction to improve people's lives. One of those nurses was Mary Breckinridge, the daughter of a distinguished Kentucky family. Her grandfather was vice president of the United States and later served as secretary of war for the Confederacy. Her father was a career diplomat who served as American minister to Russia. She volunteered in France after World War I and was impressed by the French nurse-midwives. She wanted to replicate these services for mothers and babies in her native state of Kentucky and studied midwifery herself in London. On her return, Mary met with potential and influential supporters in 1925. The Kentucky Committee for Mothers and Children was born at that meeting. She understood the importance of data collection and analysis to determine the effectiveness of the proposed service, and surveyed births and deaths in Leslie County as a baseline. She also spent that summer enlisting support from leading citizens to form the first branch committee (Wilkie & Moseley, 1969; Breckinridge, 1952).

As the service expanded, Mary Breckinridge met with insurance representatives from New York, Hartford, and Philadelphia to obtain fire insurance for the rural hospital and outposts. Metropolitan Life Insurance Company collaborated with Breckinridge to tabulate statistics and begin a health insurance program that became one of the first managed care programs in the U.S. for hospital and home care services (Judd et. al, 2010). The Carnegie Corporation helped the service accrue the only statistics of OB facts in the country, and the nurse-midwives of Frontier Nursing Service (FNS) became charter members of the American Association of Nurse Midwives when it was founded in 1928. Since there were no other nurse-midwives in the country, Mary decided it was time to provide midwifery training in the U.S. The Frontier Graduate School of Midwifery began in 1935 and was licensed by the Kentucky Board of Health in 1939 (Breckinridge, 1952).

Both Lillian Wald and Mary Breckinridge illustrate positive examples of how nurses can bridge the intersection between politics and health care to serve individuals in need. Both demonstrated political savvy in their dealings with powerful organizations, individuals, and elected officials. They never lost sight of their ultimate goal and used ongoing communication, perseverance, and data to attract others to their cause. Wald and Breckinridge began locally and changed American culture with their ideas, enthusiasm, and involvement. Both enjoyed their challenges, and their positive attitude made them leaders in health care and life.

6

POLICY CHALLENGES

The best public policy is made when you are listening to people who are going to be impacted.

—Elizabeth Dole, n.d.

Policy and politics are not interchangeable terms, but it is necessary to understand the role of both for nurses to succeed in the political process and policy development, implementation, and evaluation. As chapter 1 offered multiple definitions of politics, there are also multiple definitions of policy. Policy is frequently not the result of a single decision, but a series of decisions leading to a course of action. This aspect of decision-making makes defining policy difficult for several reasons:

1. Implementation may require multiple decisions over a long period of time beyond the initial policy-making process;
2. The series of decisions required to define the policy may make the policy vague to interpret;
3. Policies change over time and the dynamic policy process results in shifting the definitions of issues;
4. The policy does not occur in a vacuum, and it can impact or be influenced by other policies;
5. Policy decision-making must also focus on termination or succession of the policy;
6. Non-decisions that preserve the status quo and resist change must be examined; and

7. A pattern of actions over time may result in an inadvertent policy as an outcome (Hill & Varone, 2021).

Policy has been defined in various ways, from a purposeful course of action to decisions that validate values or goals and how to achieve them. Policies do not always generate change, and resistance is possible. Stages in the policy-making process are not always uniform, and feedback loops may involve the same individuals at different stages of the process. Policy development and implementation are complex. As anyone who has developed policies knows, the policy is not always clear to everyone, and conflict over a policy will result in winners and losers (Hill & Varone, 2021).

Questions to ask when considering policy development involve the steps of the policy-making process:

1. What is the problem we are attempting to solve with a policy?
   a. Can the problem be clearly defined?
   b. Is it an isolated problem that doesn't lend itself to a policy?
   c. Is it a social problem best handled outside the policy arena or a public problem?

2. How do we decide on an agenda and where do we go from here?
   a. Do we have all the information we need, or do we need more data?
   b. How do we analyze our data?
   c. Who are our stakeholders and what do they offer?
   d. What is the institutional context to consider in agenda-setting?

3. How do we formulate policy and how do we get there?
   a. How do we precisely define our objectives?
   b. What instruments and operational elements will make the policy effective?
   c. How do we involve experts and power players who will implement the policy?
   d. What funding and resources are required for implementation?
   e. What rules and procedures must be used to implement the policy?

4. How do we implement the policy?
    a. How do we resolve conflicts from the policy formulation stage?
    b. How do we identify the key players?
    c. How do we let key decisions be made by those who implement the policy?
    d. How do we negotiate and compromise with powerful groups about ongoing decisions?
    e. How do we assess responses from those affected by the policy?
    f. How do we address overall environmental factors?

5. How do we evaluate the policy and accountability?
    a. How are policy effects accurately measured?
        i. Who benefitted from the policy?
        ii. Who did not benefit from the policy?
    b. How do evaluation criteria measure the success or failure of the policy?
        i. Is the link between the objectives and the problem appropriate or relevant?
        ii. Is the link between the objectives and actual policy effects effective?
        iii. Are the policy effects and the resources (money, time, personnel) efficient?
        iv. Is the relationship between resources and administrative outputs economical? Could fewer resources have been used or could better outputs by implementers have been obtained with identical resources?
    c. How was accountability maintained?
        i. Was evidence appropriate?
        ii. Was evidence shared and open to scrutiny?
        iii. Was data open to challenge and questioning?
        iv. Were changes made that reflected dynamic policy issues if present? (Hill & Varone, 2021)

These questions are applicable to both institutional and public policy development, implementation, and evaluation. The process is not static and feedback loops may move from one area to another as questions arise. Policy does not exist in a vacuum, and one policy may be impacted by others. While this makes definition difficult, policy-making can be a stimulating, challenging opportunity to influence change at all levels.

Public policy is defined by *Legal Dictionary* as "A course of governmental action established to address the problems of society at large, rather than individual needs on a smaller scale" (Content Team, 2019). Public policy is a complex political process with many stakeholders, including "elected politicians, political party leaders, pressure groups, civil servants, publicly employed professionals, judges, non-governmental organisations, international agencies, academic experts, journalists, and even sometimes citizens who see themselves as the passive recipients of the policy" (Hill & Varone, 2021, p. 4). Policies may determine politics and vice versa, and the role of power must be considered. If nurses seek involvement in public policies, they must remember that there are winners and losers in every public policy decision. One example involves state-level policy decisions about women's reproductive health, based on 2022's Supreme Court decision to overturn Roe v. Wade. There are arguments on both sides, and nurses must understand the steps of the policy process previously discussed to examine state policies and realize that policies such as this result from interactions of different stakeholders who have separate goals, interests, and strategies. Public policy occurs in a wider political and social context that requires balance between rules and discretion. However, this is not always the case and may "distribute differential advantages and disadvantages to the parties involved, and particularly to the members of the public affected by the policy" (Hill & Varone, 2021, p. 272).

Nurses can make a positive impact on public policies as they address social challenges, advocacy, board service, and involvement in the political process as citizen voters and candidates for public office.

7

NURSING AND SOCIAL CHALLENGES

There is a social contract between society and the profession. Under its terms, society grants the professions authority over functions vital to itself and permits them considerable autonomy in the conduct of their own affairs. In return, the professions are expected to act responsibly, always mindful of the public trust. Self-regulation to assure quality and performance is at the heart of this relationship. It is the authentic hallmark of the mature profession.

—Donabedian, A. Foreword in M. Phaneul, 1976

Nurses who understand how health policy and politics inform their practice can use this knowledge to address social challenges. There is a national focus on health care, and the public involvement in health policy is increasing. As the largest group of healthcare providers, nurses are confronted with unprecedented social challenges, and their proficiency is essential to leading in public and political situations related to healthcare issues. The pandemic caused significant disruptions to care delivery across the country, but nurses continued to honor their social contract with the public to care for individuals, families, communities, and at-risk populations. Donabedian's statement delineates the responsibilities of the nursing profession and society (the public) in this social contract. Public authorization of nurses includes licensure, public support, and legal and legislative boundaries. Nurses reciprocate by providing care to those in need based on their education, expertise, and clinical and professional judgment (ANA, 2010).

Nursing practice is regulated by state nurse practice acts, standards of practice, the code of ethics, and practice-setting policies and procedures. Such policies and procedures reflect accreditation and federal, state, or local regulations. The ultimate health outcome of this regulation is quality and safety. The American Nurses Association's *Code of Ethics for Nurses* and *Nursing Scope and Standards of Practice* are dynamic documents that are reviewed and revised as nursing and its social context change (ANA, 2015 & ANA, 2021).

The American Nurses Association (ANA) is considered the national voice for nursing, although many nurses do not belong to the organization and prefer joining their specialty organizations instead. ANA began in 1911 to succeed the Nurses Associated Alumnae of the United States. Its predecessor was the first nursing organization in the U.S. and Canada but was unable to organize nurses as they became more mobile. As ANA membership evolved via state nurses' associations, the organization used this relationship to gain legal regulation and licensing laws (Donahue, 2010).

ANA is recognized today for its representation of nurses and healthcare issues nationally. In addition to promoting high standards of practice and establishing a code of ethics for nurses, the American Nurses Association lobbies Congress and regulatory agencies about healthcare issues that affect the profession and the public. Part of its role is helping nurses everywhere address social challenges that include health policy and regulation (ANA, 2010).

According to ANA, nurses have an active leadership role in political and public venues about six key healthcare areas:

- Quality health care: Nurses must address how to reduce healthcare costs and health disparities while ensuring accessible, safe, and available healthcare resources and services;
- Public health services: Nurses must share information about disease prevention, health promotion, and environmental actions with the public, including self-help measures;
- Growth of healthcare knowledge and use of technology: Nurses must incorporate evidence and research in practice to generate and apply knowledge and technology to health outcomes;
- Health policy and healthcare resources: Nurses must support expansion of community health services to promote self-help and self-care for individuals and populations;

- Health policy planning and regulation: Nurses must collaborate to respond to needs of consumers and assure the best use of resources to provide health care for everyone; and
- Duties in extreme emergencies: Nurses must weigh their own health and that of their families with their duty to provide care under extreme conditions (ANA, 2010).

These six social concerns are evident in today's nursing practice as well as in nurses' private lives. Nursing is not separate from society. Nurses are affected by societal issues along with other citizens. This is reflected in the *American Journal of Nursing* column about the top social justice issues in 2022, which include in no particular order:

- Gun violence resulting in increased levels of homicide and suicide by firearms of 8.3% since 2020 with most deaths in Black or African American individuals;
- Women's reproductive health abortion bans in some states following the overturn of Roe v. Wade including legal penalties for healthcare providers providing abortion care;
- Racism in health care being addressed with diversity, equity, and inclusion initiatives that acknowledge systemic racism and implicit bias while implementing antiracist programs;
- Crisis on the border resulting in more than 2 million immigrants at the border without a clear plan to address the influx;
- Antitransgender legislation in some state legislatures that include restrictions on sports participation and medical care that is gender-affirming; and
- War in Ukraine resulting in large refugee displacement and human rights violations (Szukecki, 2023, pp. 14–15).

These hot-button issues defy easy solutions because nurses and other citizens espouse strong beliefs about some and not others. Nurses must understand that their beliefs may or may not be held by others, including their peers. Understanding beliefs is probably the most difficult aspect of social justice challenges to acknowledge, and the most important to know. Bi-directional communication and collaboration are essential if we are to receive true social justice where everyone has equal rights and opportunities. To achieve true collaboration, all parties must respect and understand others viewpoints to accomplish common goals. True collaboration requires trust and recognition of each person's contributions by developing relationships with diverse individuals who bring a different perspective to the issues (ANA, 2010).

Social justice issues are challenges where nurses have expertise and can make a positive difference locally and regionally, particularly in the policy arena. Our current health system is in crisis. Healthcare costs are rising, causing many individuals to decline essential care due to increasing costs and lack of coverage for expensive treatments to treat major illnesses (e.g., chemotherapy, thrombolytics, antidepressants). Chronic diseases (e.g., diabetes, heart disease, depression) are increasing, and inequities continue to affect poor and disadvantaged populations. Social determinants of health (SDOH) are major factors in health inequities "that are a result of systemic, avoidable and unjust social and economic policies and practices that create barriers to opportunity" (Rudolph et al., 2013, p. 9).

Health inequities differ from health disparities, and it is important to understand the difference. Health disparities are health differences based on race, gender, age, ethnicity, or geographic location. Some of these, such as sickle cell or Tay Sachs disease, are not responsive to changes in policies or practices. Other disparities, such as lead poisoning in children living in outdated buildings, are responsive to eradication policies of lead-based paint in such residences. Policy focusing on health inequities can improve some disparities while addressing social, economic, and environmental issues (apha.org, 2018).

Addressing social challenges requires concerted efforts and cannot succeed alone. It takes a village of collaborators working together to make progress toward health equity where everyone can thrive. Health equity requires responsible management of resources and stewardship to sustain social, environmental, and economic results now and in the future. Stakeholders who will be affected by the results must be involved in the process. They may be academic experts, private sector and non-governmental organizations, community-based organizations and members, private sector companies, and funders. Private sector companies can provide essential resources, and funders can allocate funds to support stakeholder engagement. Stakeholders' engagement has numerous advantages, including

- increased community action;
- more support for health policies and programs affecting the community;
- improved relationships between members of the above sectors;

- better understanding about the roles of local, regional, state, and federal government agencies and how their policies and programs affect community well-being and health;
- enhanced knowledge about social determinants of health;
- better involvement of community members in government processes; and
- improved communication with policymakers (Rudolph et al., 2013).

Nurses are community members as well as professionals. As members of the most trusted profession, they can play a significant role in addressing social challenges (Advisory Board, 2023 & ana.org, 2023). Collaboration requires trust to build relationships between partners from multiple sectors. Everyone must be open to learning from each other and acknowledge that there will be differences in opinions. Open-minded listening, transparency, and accountability are traits to cultivate. Confidentiality must also be respected in sensitive discussions. Everyone must honor their commitments and offer support as needed. Giving credit to other partners for their contributions will make them more likely to engage in collaborative solutions. Aligning values and goals will keep everyone on the same page, resulting in shared vision and win-win opportunities when addressing social challenges (Rudolph et al., 2013).

There is never assurance that results will meet everyone's expectations, but by working together the team can make progress toward the final goal—where everyone has equal rights and opportunities to achieve health equity (apha.org, 2018).

8

NURSES AS ADVOCATES

I alone cannot change the world, but I can cast a stone across the waters to create many ripples.

—Mother Teresa, n.d.

Mother Teresa's words describe the ripple effect of advocacy. The term is often interpreted narrowly when in reality its scope is broad. Nurses are obligated to advocate for the individuals and populations they serve, but they can also advocate for local, regional, national, and global issues. As defined in the *Code of Ethics for Nurses,* advocacy is "The act or process of pleading for, supporting, or recommending a cause or course of action. Advocacy may be for persons (whether as an individual, group, population, or society) or for an issue, such as potable water or global health" (ANA, 2015, p. 41).

With this definition in mind, what competencies are essential to be a true advocate? A nurse advocate demonstrates the following skills:

- champions the voice of the healthcare consumer;
- promotes safe care, safe work environments, and resource allocation to optimize outcomes;
- participates in initiatives to benefit the healthcare consumer;
- addresses pervasive, persistent systemic issues;
- promotes the role of nurses and requirements for optimal care delivery to political leaders;
- ensures the healthcare consumer is included in all decisions for his or her care;

- embraces diversity, equity, and inclusion in health care and health promotion for individuals and populations;
- develops policies to improve care delivery and access for vulnerable, underserved populations;
- promotes policies, legislation, and regulations at local, state, and national levels to improve access and delivery of health care;
- addresses social determinants of health by considering political, economic, societal, and cultural factors;
- confronts the need for an inclusive and diverse workforce to improve health outcomes;
- advances programs, policies, and practices to maintain, sustain, and restore the environment; and
- contributes to professional organizations as a role model for advocacy (ANA, 2021).

With these skills in mind, an advocate requires three essential qualities: planning, persistence, and passion. Advocacy on an issue is not a spur of the moment activity. True advocacy requires careful planning and starts with researching the issue. Nurses use evidence in practice, and it is equally important for advocacy. No one can be an effective advocate without carefully investigating all aspects of the issue. When planning has occurred, the advocate must remember that results will not occur instantly or even at all. Persistence is required for any chance of success in the short or long term. Obstacles and roadblocks will occur and how the advocate handles these setbacks is indicative of how successful the initiative and the advocate will be now and in the future. Passion is fuel for advocacy. If an advocate is not passionate about the issue at hand, momentum will falter, and the disillusioned advocate will move on to other issues or causes.

It also helps to have the support of like-minded individuals. The saying "it takes a village" is true of advocacy. Working with dedicated partners will help the advocate stay focused on the road ahead. It's easy to get discouraged when you are alone. Support from others can make the struggle easier and the results more positive. An example of group advocacy is the American Nurses Association Political Action Center (ANA PAC). The purpose of ANA PAC is to ensure that nurses have a voice in national politics and to elect nurse champions to Congress. Since the American Nurses Association and similar organizations are prohibited by federal law from endorsing or contributing to national political candidates, this separate arm of the organization was established to support national candidates who champion ANA's legislative priorities and is solely funded by individual members' contributions (ANA, 2022).

ANA PAC supports Congressional candidates who will address problems affecting nurses like safe staffing and affordable access to care. Funding by individual nurses enables nurses to be involved in healthcare issues and have a voice in government beyond voting in elections. Endorsement may be with or without monetary funding. Candidates are carefully screened, and incumbents' voting records are scrutinized to ensure that they reflect advocacy for nursing and health care. As a nonpartisan PAC, ANA PAC endorses candidates of all political parties and focuses its efforts on both houses of Congress. Member dues are not used to fund ANA PAC. Contributions are voluntary and not tax deductible. Each nurse decides whether or not to contribute and membership in ANA does not require any contribution to ANA PAC. If a nurse desires to contribute, he or she decides the amount and frequency of contributions. Policymakers in Congress recognize ANA as the voice of nursing nationally and the ANA PAC must represent the interests of all 4.3 million nurses in the United States in their activities (ANA, 2022).

ANA PAC is administered by a Board of 11 trustees. Three members are appointed by the ANA President and are also serving on the ANA Board of Directors (BOD). Eight members are appointed by the ANA BOD based on the recommendation of the Committee on Appointments. Members must be active ANA members, registered voters, contributors to ANA PAC, have fundraising capability, and have involvement in political activities and lobbying at local, state, or national levels (ANA, 2022).

Within ANA PAC is the Leadership Society, comprised currently of 14 members who are leaders of political activism with extraordinary political skill and talent. These individuals are selected by the ANA PAC Board of Trustees and exemplify the relationship between nursing, policy, politics, and ANA PAC. These fellows remain in the Leadership Society as long as they are active ANA members and committed to political activism (ANA, 2022).

Here are some of their stories.

> Elizabeth's journey to advocacy with ANA PAC started when she decided to self-nominate for a director position in ANA and won! She spent the first year of her term learning from ANA leaders and then was asked to select a committee in

the organization. She chose ANA PAC and was mentored by the ANA PAC chair and co-founder of the Leadership Society. After her term on ANA PAC, Elizabeth moved to the Leadership Society to continue her advocacy work. The Leadership Society members support annual goals, current education, fundraising, and mobilization of nurses. She also works with her students to develop nursing-specific toolkits to mobilize nurses to speak out on healthcare issues at all levels. There is not a game plan at the PAC to engage nurses' involvement at the local level. She encourages her students to identify what they are most passionate about and encourages them to volunteer as members of their policy and procedure committee to gain leadership experience and move forward into the chair role. These committees are safe places to move issues forward and address issues that will become policies at their organization. This experience can help them move issues forward at other levels: local, state, and even national. Elizabeth is also a recognized tobacco control expert who started a single help line that evolved into a program with over $10 million in grants. Her opportunity to serve on state commissions and boards allowed her to meet advocates who shared her passion, and they were successful in passing state tobacco prevention legislation. She believes it is vital to be surrounded by people who are equally passionate about issues because advocacy is sometimes an arduous process, and nurturing each other is essential. On the state level, she is collaborating with other nurses, nursing students, and legislators to introduce a bill for nursing compact legislation. Elizabeth encourages her colleagues and students to share stories because stories make individuals memorable. She believes that advocates must be transparent and have integrity in relationships. To be an effective advocate, a nurse must be trusted and understand how to check his or her ego to be able to listen to others' viewpoints and compromise to support the common issue. She believes letting go of her own ego to support decisions is vital to success. In her words "The sign of emotional intelligence is the ability to compromise" (Fildes, 2023).

Gayle was a staff nurse at a large east coast facility for her entire career, but her involvement in advocacy started in local politics and continues to this day. Gayle worked with the Leukemia Society in college and attended meetings with legislators to advocate for cancer legislation. She learned how to interact with political leaders and their staff members about important issues in health care. Subsequently, she participated in an internship in Washington, DC and her enthusiasm led her to staff leadership positions within her organization and region as chairperson of the organization's Ethics Committee and chairperson of the American Society of Pain Management Nursing (ASPMN) in her state. Gayle also served as staff nurse representative on the ANA board of directors and was appointed to ANA PAC where she served as co-chairperson of the group. At the time, the ANA PAC Leadership Society was dormant, and she and her co-chairperson contacted former society leaders for ideas to rejuvenate the group. Their efforts were successful, and the Leadership Society is still functional today. Gayle stresses that ANA PAC is the decision-making body and support is bipartisan for those who support nursing legislation. Society members are role models for advocacy individually.

Gayle's career focused on ethics and pain management as a senior nurse on an in-patient oncology unit, and she continues to successfully advocate for policy legislation. Her advocacy includes the passage of a bill for sunscreen on beaches, and for students to apply sunscreen without it being considered medication. She has worked in legislative campaigns and continues her access to legislators regarding healthcare issues. She has served on the Safe Staffing Task Force for her state's hospital association as the only staff nurse present, and the only member who has worked with patients in the past 5 years. As she said, "Think tanks have ideas, but don't go to staff nurses for input" (Peterson, 2023).

Gayle shared why staff nurses are not more involved in legislative advocacy. Many of these nurses join specialty organizations, not the ANA, because they don't relate to the ANA and its activities. Staff nurses lack time to study issues impacting their patients and their practice. Even if staff nurses want to participate in the legislative process, bills in committees have hearings with only 1 to 2 days' notice. Staff nurses don't have time to get off work, travel to the Statehouse, and testify. Colleagues and managers must keep staff nurses informed about issues, listen to staff nurses, and enable them to participate in legislative advocacy.

Gayle's advice to today's practicing nurses, educators, and student is

- õ Find out who your legislators are and their positions;
- õ Share stories in discussion with legislators and staff and testimony (stories are powerful);
- õ Encourage the inclusion of courses course in nursing programs about nursing policy and advocacy so students will know how the legislative process works;
- õ Encourage participation in Hill Days; and
- õ Partner with students in addressing legislative healthcare issues (Peterson, 2023).

Liz's road to advocacy was different. She realized that advocacy was something important when she passed her Boards. After that, she joined the USPHS (United States Public Health Service) in Massachusetts and joined the Massachusetts Nurses Association and ANA. Initially, she followed information and wrote letters supporting positions. Her advocacy grew over the years, and she has been active in ANA and state nurses associations everywhere she has lived and practiced. Although community health is her specialty, Liz has taught childbirth classes and OB in the university setting. She has held numerous roles in ANA including two terms on the board of directors, the Reference Committee, Nursing Practice Committee, and Nursing Finance Committee. Currently, she is co-chairperson of the Committee on Nursing Practice Standards. She joined ANA PAC when appointed by the ANA board and served several years. Her advocacy skills grew from attending conventions and Hill visits as well as serving as a volunteer lobbyist (Dietz, 2023).

Liz is active in the ANA PAC Leadership Society to support the PAC, board of directors, and legislative issues. She has always donated to ANA PAC and encourages other nurses "to open their pockets and contribute." Her enthusiasm is obvious, and she says serving on ANA PAC has been fun! She has met Rosalyn Carter and has a picture of Corretta Scott King and her at a PAC event. Although some politicians believe ANA only supports one political party, Liz is adamant that party affiliation is unimportant if the legislator supports nursing issues. She believes politics is important in nursing education and exists in all organizations, including nonprofits and service agencies. Nurse educators and leaders could take the following actions to ensure that political issues impacting practice are included in formal and informal education: include a session on politics in annual organization conferences; promote changing the NCLEX to include current healthcare issues instead of only teaching the illness and disease model; and change the framework of nursing education to address topical political issues in multiple clinical areas (e.g., -OB-WIC, food stamps, abortion) instead of just one course.

Liz's advice for nurses considering a role in advocacy is

- õ Begin by understanding the politics in your state; how you get legislation passed and how does legislation become regulation;
- õ Understand that the political process is important material for nursing education programs and state nurses' associations;
- õ Understand participation in social media and do it properly;
- õ Don't sit idly by;
- õ Consider stepping up and running for office; and
- õ Become part of the team of legislators as a health expert. All you need to do is call the legislator's office and say "I live and voted in your district. I am a nurse." They will welcome you (Deitz, 2023).

Enjoy the challenge of advocacy and have fun!

9

NURSES ON BOARDS

A wise board accumulates rational wisdom, embraces unconventional wisdom and sharpens system wisdom.

—Pearl Zhu, n.d.

Board service is an excellent way to be involved in decision-making groups that affect nurses, consumers, and families. As with advocacy, the first step is often the most difficult. Luckily, there are resources for nurses who want to serve on boards but don't know how to go about it or what serving entails. The Nurses on Boards Coalition (NOBC) is an excellent resource for nurses seeking board service. The NOBC is the result of a nationwide effort by the AARP (American Association of Retired Persons) Foundation and the Robert Wood Johnson Foundation in 2014. The mission was to increase the number of nurses in decision-making positions on boards and commissions working to improve health equity for all citizens. Their initial goal was to ensure that nurses filled at least 10,000 board seats by 2020. After achieving that goal, NOBC now measures the impact of these nurses on boards and raises awareness of how all boards would benefit from the presence and perspective of nurses to improve health and healthcare systems at all levels (NOBC, 2022).

NOBC has three strategies for 2022–2025. These include board placements for nurses:

- to influence policies in the community that ensure equity and social justice;
- that measure success related to desired outcomes; and
- that reflect NOBC core work in board appointments (NOBC, 2022).

Nonprofit and corporate board opportunities are available and NOBC ensures that nurses applying for these boards are ready and qualified to serve. The initial step in board service is to focus on organizations and causes that feed your passion. If the topics and issues involved aren't inspiring, it will be difficult to stay interested in the results. Nurses seeking board opportunities must begin by carefully assessing their own preferences. Once that has occurred and the selected board has an opening, the next step is skills assessment. How do your skills fit with the organization's mission, vision, and values? NOBC has a Readiness Assessment for Board Service that highlights seven leadership competencies for board participation. The assessment tool is designed for personal use and indicates self-scoring for competencies of governance, leadership, relationship building and collaboration, inspiring others, adaptability, communication skills, and engagement. It is an opportunity to review strengths and areas for improvement.

What's next? It's time to develop skills that will set you up for success in board service. Formal and informal education are available to become the candidate the board wants as a member. Start by outlining your strengths for board service using the board core competencies.

1. **Mission**: You are committed to advancing the organization's mission as a framework for decisions.
2. **Communication**: You communicate effectively, professionally, confidently, and calmly; listen respectfully; focus on facts; and are comfortable with challenge and inquiry.
3. **Cultural awareness and competence**: You initiate and support board actions to promote diversity, equity, and inclusion where everyone is treated fairly and respectfully, their worth and dignity is recognized, and all have access to opportunities.
4. **Leadership**: You have the skills, knowledge, and attitude to lead others and demonstrate systems thinking by focusing on the big picture, relationships, and connections between parts and services (NOBC, 2022).

One area is missing from the above list of strengths—financial knowledge. Imagine this is the board core competency that you realize needs improvement from your self-assessment. You have monitored your own financial budgets and can read and understand a balance sheet and income statement. However, you have limited knowledge of audits and tax requirements, particularly as they impact the organization represented by the board. Fortunately, there are resources to help you learn this information. Seek them out and ask an experienced board member to guide you in attaining this knowledge. Remember, you are not expected to know everything in the beginning, but you are expected to be honest about areas of improvement and to seek resources to enhance your skillset (NOBC, 2022).

As your financial skills increase, you will be able to review and approve budgets, compare actual and projected figures, verify that variances can be explained and rectified, and understand the audit process and the board's role in reviewing Form 990 for tax-exempt organizations. Once you gain these skills, you and your fellow board members can partner with the organization's staff to develop and evaluate the organization's direction and goals through strategic oversight. Finally, board members and the CEO must use generative insight to analyze and discuss issues using critical thinking and debate to focus on long-term priorities related to the mission and goals.

Generative governance is not a quick fix. It requires a commitment from everyone in preparation for meetings, and changes in how those meetings are structured. Generative governance includes:

1. Pre-reading by board members so everyone comes prepared to share their ideas;
2. Use of a consent agenda to streamline review of reports and project approval;
3. A meeting agenda created by the CEO and board chair to ensure time to discuss and analyze critical issues with the most important items and any related items first;
4. Questions that are open-ended, relate to the mission and goals, and focus on long-term priorities; and
5. Everyone's voice is heard and new ways of analyzing ideas and big-picture questions are encouraged (NOBC, 2022).

Since critical thinking is essential to success in generative governance, barriers must be addressed. These include:

- Fearing being wrong or falling prey to groupthink;
- Differentiating between a "gut feeling" and information supported by data;
- Having an initial assumption or conclusion and assuming everyone agrees on the solution; and
- Assuming board members always make rational decisions (NOBC, 2022).

Addressing these barriers requires multiple approaches such as:

- Encourage questions, not statements, and use small groups to discuss different solutions in discussions;
- Have board members play devil's advocate and approach a question from a different perspective;
- Ask board members to write down the most important question they think should be considered before discussing an issue. Then anonymously read these responses and tally all similar questions; and
- Focus on how decisions are made and on opportunities, not problems (NOBC, 2022).

Generative governance may lead to higher-level thinking, more effective and engaging board meetings, and a stronger organization. However, it is important to realize that every organization and board may not be ready to implement generative governance. The leadership model must serve the purpose of the organization and generative governance may be a future goal to identify innovative solutions that advance the mission when the board and leadership are ready to evolve to it (NOBC, 2022).

With this background in mind, let's hear from some nurses about their board service. Flora, Sarah, Rachel, and Karen are experienced board members on the local, regional, and national levels who are willing to share their experiences here.

1. What preparation did you have before joining your first board?
    a. "My position as Emergency Services director afforded me opportunities to participate in various work groups of diverse leadership. Often times the diversity of these groups included areas of the operations I was not familiar with, yet needed to collaborate to achieve departmental goals. The yin and yang of these work groups were strong examples of the need for superior communication and mediation to achieve the group's goals, often seen on board activities." —Flora
    b. "Served 15 years on the Board of Directors of Cancer Services regionally and represented nursing and the university as a nursing professor. Member of the Board of Trustees (Neuman Systems Model [NSM] Trustees, Inc.) where my experience from the previous board helped prepare me." —Sarah

c. "I don't feel that I had any purposeful preparation for board service. As a bedside nurse, I was not actively engaged in my professional organizations and did not sit on any committees for my workplace. So, the idea of being on a board never even entered my mind. I thought board appointments were for wealthy folks or experts with something important to offer (I did not consider myself any of those things!). In graduate school, I was inducted into Sigma. Shortly after joining, I was asked to consider filling a vacancy in the Governance committee. I didn't even know what the word Governance meant, let alone what the committee work would entail. The only reason I agreed to the role was because there were already two experienced members on that committee who were willing to teach me. This 'gentle' introduction was beneficial, because it didn't overwhelm me and gave me a chance to see that I could belong on a board. Over time, I took on different roles and joined other committees, which significantly expanded my understanding of board service. Looking back, I think my work as a faculty member did help me understand some things about board service. Participating on committees, navigating budget and accreditation issues, being involved with policy and programmatic decision-making were all relevant to the experiences I would later encounter on the board. However, I feel most of my learning has been through 'hands-on' experience while actively serving on boards." —Rachel

d. "My first board role was on the Washington State Chapter of the Cystic Fibrosis Foundation. My preparation was only as a parent of a child with cystic fibrosis. I had experience with the disease but not really the business aspects of the foundation so I had to learn the balance sheet of the chapter, marketing plan, and community outreach. I did have familiarity with the local clinical care resources." —Karen

2. Did you have a mentor for board service?

   a. "At an early point in my employment, the vice president of nursing encouraged me to seek board work and was instrumental in mentoring me. Her guidance focused on not only my skills, but also how the board (or executive work group) would benefit from my participation. She was always accessible for problem-solving when needed and redirection when warranted." —Flora

b. "No mentor for the Cancer Services Board and yes, an experienced & renowned Trustee as mentor for NSM." —Sarah

c. "Yes. The person who encouraged me to take my first board position served as a mentor. However, that relationship was established prior to me joining the board. Had that person not already been a part of my life, I (a) probably wouldn't have joined the board, but also (b) wouldn't have received any mentorship during my initial years of board service. As I've taken on other roles within that board and joined other boards, I do not feel I've had any mentorship. It has been my experience that people are always willing to help me learn, but that help usually results from me reaching out. It is not a proactive or thoughtful process of mentorship. Unfortunately, I don't think I've been much of a mentor to others who are beginning their board service either." —Rachel

d. "I never had a formal mentor, but I did ask a number of questions of those who had more knowledge than I and would seek to speak with a colleague prior to the meeting depending on the agenda items. As I served on other boards, I became more versant with the role of board member and was comfortable asking questions. I also became more knowledgeable about meeting rules. I believe (in retrospect) that understanding the dynamics of how a meeting is conducted is just as essential as content." —Karen

3. How do you evaluate board opportunities?

   a. "The first thing I assess is the purpose/goals of the board. Are they consistent with my philosophy? For me to be successful and the board to benefit from my participation, compatible philosophy, process thinking and strategic goals are critical. Next, I examine my motives for seeking to join the board. Am I motivated to lead or participate? Can I be effective without being 'in-charge'? I compare the role qualifications and ensure that I meet them without modification. I ask myself if I have the time and energy bandwidth to do the job as it deserves. I examine the board to determine if its goals and methods are in conflict with any of my other volunteer roles. Or are they in fact synergistic? Finally, I inquire if the board is a fiduciary one, expecting a donation—and is that feasible?" —Flora

b. "I am often recruited for my expertise in select areas such as: leadership as an officer, educational offerings, and chair of planning committee. Fundraising is a given, must learn how to do the ask." —Sarah

c. "Before serving on a board, I didn't have any framework for evaluating board opportunities. Now that I've spent time serving on a few, I have a better understanding of what opportunities might be a good fit. I am no longer naïve about the commitments that a board position can entail. In my current phase of life, the time commitment is a major factor in my decision to join a board. When you join a board, people will not only expect you to do your part, they are counting on it. So, if I do not have the availability or energy to fulfill those expectations, I should not accept them. I also consider whether the board position is a good fit for my skill set. Like the rationale above, I need to be able to do my part. If I don't have the skills and abilities needed for the role, I should not pursue it. I also consider whether the organization aligns with my values. If I were involved in a board that didn't excite me or work toward goals that matter to me, my heart would not be in the service." —Rachel

d. "1) Do I believe I have expertise and experience to add value to the organization? 2) What is the time requirement both in week/month and expected number of years that the organization expects? 3) Is the mission of the organization consistent with my values and belief system?" —Karen

4. What skills do you bring to a board?

   a. "My skills in written and verbal communication are the strongest assets I bring to any board or organization. My skills in this regard have been honed by multiple publications and presentation opportunities. I have the education, experience, and skill in Human Resource Management and therefore bring an appreciation of the value of diverse thinking and respect for others. I have a sense of humor, applied in the appropriate setting, to be a force of light and pleasantness. I have strong skills in data (statistical) and narrative information analysis." —Flora

b. "My skills include leadership, confidence, team builder, treasurer, president, and recruitment." —Sarah
c. "I am not great at tooting my own horn, but I think these are some skills and qualities that I bring to the table:

   i. Enthusiasm and eagerness to support the board's success.
   ii. I'm pretty savvy with technology and willing to learn new tools, which has proved useful for a variety of reasons. I can and have developed electronic surveys, managed social media and website platforms, and used web conferencing, streaming, and sharing services (Google Drive, You Tube) to support the board's goals and activities.
   iii. I like to be very respectful of other people's time, so I tend to be prepared and focused during meetings.
   iv. Openness to new ideas.
   v. Willingness to learn.
   vi. A nursing perspective (particularly relevant for non-nursing organizations).
   vii. Knowledge about course design and accessibility." —Rachel

d. "My strengths include working in a number of different areas and many different organizations. In nursing, I have been a staff RN, Charge RN, Case Manager, Clinical Nurse Specialist and Director/Administrator and Consultant roles of Lead, Principal and Executive Consultant. My work has taken me into more organizations than most and the nature of my consulting work required that I learn about the organization as I was recommending changes to take them to the desired future state. I am a systems thinker and able to synthesize information quickly so that I can organize the work that I must do and meet the timelines. When employed in a single organization, I asked to do additional assignments as time permitted to keep the work challenging. My experience in quality and measurement has been an asset to me." —Karen

5. What have you learned from board service?

   a. "I have learned to evaluate opinions that differ from me and be comfortable with 'meeting in the middle'. I am less rigid in my opinions and approaches to problem-solving. I have also learned to step away from a board if and when I no longer can contribute at the level, I set myself, without feeling like a failure." —Flora

b. "Board service is service–not paid–one must want to do this. It requires effort, input, time, and energy. I found my contributions were consistently appreciated which was rewarding. To serve was an honor. I learned new and creative fundraising strategies." —Sarah
c. "Leadership: This is an area I have always struggled with and continually strive to grow in. My board positions have forced me to step up and lead in different ways that stretch my skills and help me gain confidence.

    i. Strategic Planning. This concept was like a buzzword to me, but I have learned that understanding your Mission and Vision matter, and that you have to have alignment between these things and your activities to continue forward progress.
    ii. Delegation.
    iii. Collaboration skills.
    iv. The value of networking, and a bit about how to do it (still growing in this area!).
    v. Outreach and public relations.
    vi. Fundraising." —Rachel

d. "Some organizations are truly transparent and interested in achieving goals and moving forward; some, not so much. It is important to understand the culture before challenging the status quo. Always seek to understand and listen to other points of view. Agree to disagree, but always be respectful of others with different viewpoints. Learn where the organization is what they value (this may be different from stated goals)." —Karen

6. What advice do you have for nurses seeking board service?

    a. "Start with examining the goals of the board and ask yourself if these goals fire your passion. What is your knowledge regarding the mission of the organization the board represents? Be honest with yourself about time, energy and financial commitment. If the opportunity presents itself, can you attend a meeting prior to officially joining? If yes, watch carefully the interpersonal dynamics as opposed to the policies and practices. Are these individuals you want to work with? Are these individuals you want to learn from? Definitely seek a mentor who will objectively assess your motives and skills and guide you toward success." —Flora

b. "Evaluate your interests. Seek board service that taps your expertise and skillset. Be proud of the work and contributions you give, in other words, give it your best. Be alert to your own time available to give of self—if you must step down due to unforeseen reasons, it is OK. Help recruit a qualified replacement for consideration." —Sarah
c. "First and foremost, I recommend that nurses focus on service that is aligned with their interests, expertise, and/or passions. It can be extremely rewarding and motivating when your service helps generate outcomes that are personally meaningful. When your purpose aligns with that of your board, service feels like a blessing you want to make time for, rather than a burden you must make time for. Similarly, the position should fit with their skill set (even if it stretches them a bit) so they can feel good about their contributions and like a valued member of the board. I also encourage nurses to start in a comfortable role where they can learn about the nature of the board, including its purpose and functions, and what is expected of them. As they engage in low-stakes learning opportunities (e.g., attending board meetings, contributing to projects, etc.), they will develop a more complete understanding of their roles, gain confidence in their ability to contribute, and begin accepting more responsibility or new roles. Similarly, I would warn against accepting too much responsibility. When seeking or accepting a board appointment, a nurse should be very clear about their availability and boundaries." —Rachel
d. "Be authentic and represent yourself as such. Understand the need to spend time learning the foundation of the organization—bylaws, policies, budgetary information, etc. Build partnerships with those on the board. Seek to understand the environment in which the organization operates—regulatory, financial, and human resources as a background for meaningful forward movement. Stay abreast of trends and any events or legislation that may impact the organization." —Karen

Hopefully, the experience and advice of these nurses on the topic of board service will resonate with anyone interested in joining and contributing to a local board.

Boards also advocate with legislators about issues of importance and advancing causes that the organization supports. This chapter would be incomplete without addressing this aspect of board service. Preparation beforehand is essential. Board members must:

- Understand how public policy affects your ability to serve residents in the community based on your mission and programs;
- Examine local, state, and federal public policy proposals that could harm or advance your mission;
- Acquaint yourself with individuals leading policy development and implementation;
- Strategically target legislators and inform them about your organization's work in the community;
- Identify the most appropriate board members to form relationships with legislators based on community standing, personality, or career role; and
- Seek a meeting with the selected legislator starting with a formal email, a follow-up phone call, or making an appointment in person (NOBC, 2022).

Remember that a request for a 30-minute meeting may only be awarded 15 minutes with a legislator. Now that the meeting is scheduled, the selected board members must be prepared to quickly and succinctly present information about the organization's impact and how this reflects the legislator's interests. Your ask must be clear for the legislator to grasp your expectations, and you should get to the point promptly.

It's a good idea to have a more experienced board member advise you about how to tailor your presentation when discussing the organization's work and accomplishments. It helps to rehearse beforehand to refine your talking points. Building positive relationships with the legislator and key staff members will begin with the first interactions and takes time. Begin by establishing a good foundation in the first meeting. Don't forget the importance of staffers who can support your positions within the legislator's interests and newly elected or minority party legislators who can be allies later on.

Check out the legislator's policy positions, voting history, biography, and personal website. The meeting should include no more than three to four people and one will be the principal spokesperson. These may include a staff policy person from the organization, a member of the community served, and a constituent from the legislator's district (preferably the spokesperson). Stories are powerful when they tie the legislator's interests or past votes to your issue or cause (NOBC, 2022).

As the meeting ends, ask if the legislator has any questions or needs further clarification and reinforce the best way to contact her or him. Be sure to provide any requested additional information promptly and always write a thank-you note. Hopefully, this initial meeting will be the first of many.

There are specific legal guidelines that boards must follow based on specific types of organizations. Boards may advocate for broad topics related to educational meetings, educational materials, and educating policymakers about public policy issues. However, 501(c)(3) organizations may engage in lobbying to influence legislation as long as this does not constitute a substantial part of its overall activities. If this occurs, the organization risks losing its tax-exempt status, and this is determined by such factors as the time and expenditures spent by the organization in this activity. *Substantial* is not clearly defined by the IRS, so organizations must be careful when engaging in lobbying efforts. Private foundations are generally prohibited from lobbying because they incur an excise tax on these expenditures (IRS, 2022). When in doubt, the board should refer to tax information and resources for clarification.

The Stand for Your Mission website is an excellent resource for board members to be actively engaged as advocates for their organization's work. Public policy impacts organization strategy, and advocating for the mission is part of each board member's roles and responsibilities. Board members can use their passion and influence in the community to help legislators and officials realize that their decisions can accelerate your impact on the public that you all serve. Lastly, engaging in advocacy as a board member doesn't require a major time commitment. Besides meeting with a legislator, you can call someone to ensure that your organization can connect with the right decision-maker. If you are having an educational meeting, invite decision-makers to attend and learn more about your organization's role. Focus on how you can partner with leaders and policymakers to serve their stakeholders and yours (boardsource.org, 2020).

That's a win-win-win!

10

FOSTERING NURSES' POLITICAL AWARENESS

Is nursing ready to take on a role as a pathfinder or trendsetter and engage in anticipatory nursing or are its members waiting for directions given by other disciplines who are often less well equipped to act as a liaison between policy-makers and planners of care and the public at large?

—Hanneke van Maanen, MA, RN,
1990 cited in Donahue, 2010

Awareness about the steps of the policymaking process is essential when nurses anticipate their involvement as pathfinders and trendsetters in today's complex healthcare environment. However, Maanen's quote must be addressed if nurses are to become today's change agents. The life and accomplishments of another American nurse named Lavinia Lloyd Dock may answer the question, "Is nursing ready?" Lavinia Dock was a pathfinder and trendsetter during a time when women were not considered equal citizens. In the first quarter of the twentieth century, she actively supported unions and the women's suffrage movement. Her work in supporting the union movement for workers and advocating for women's right to vote caused her to be arrested three times for picketing. Miss Dock also crusaded to secure laws for nursing control over the profession to "establish a recognized standard of professional nursing" (Dock, 1900). She achieved her goal for women's rights with the adoption of the Nineteenth Amendment on August 18, 1920: "The right of citizens of the United States to vote shall not be denied or abridged by the United States or by any state on account of sex. Congress shall have power to enforce this article by appropriate legislation" (U.S. Const. amend. XIX).

The right to vote was an opportunity for nurses (who are a part of a primarily women's profession) to become involved in the political process on local, regional, and national levels. Voting enabled them to assess and support candidates who shared their viewpoints on issues. Then and now nurses are individuals who make their own decisions about policy and political involvement. Their knowledge of health care, social determinants of health, and the impact of policies and politics on communities and underserved populations make them valuable voters and citizens.

However, many nurses are reluctant to become politically active and are unsure of how they can navigate and impact the current political process. The first step is political awareness, and this requires education and practice. There are resources available, and some begin with basic voting skills.

The American Nurses Association (ANA) has an RNAction site that provides information about current national nursing priorities. It also can help nurses with their voter registration status and provide information about elected officials and candidates in their area of residence. The site also includes information about how to get involved locally. This includes holding a voter registration drive; signing up for a phone or text bank shift; volunteering for a candidate or at a polling center; visiting a town hall or campaign event locally; connecting with state nurses' association leaders; getting out the vote and using resources from the RNAction website. These resources may include registered nurse or registered voter buttons and a free Healthy Democracy Kit from Vot-ER to promote voter registration. These resources are public information for nurses (ANA, 2023).

After increased voting knowledge, nurses can expand their political competence by attending advocacy programs and meetings sponsored by state nurses' associations. The Minnesota Organization of Registered Nurses has an annual program for nurses from any state nurses' association to develop their political awareness and competency called The American Nurses Advocacy Institute. More than 108 nurses from 36 states have participated in this program since its inception. Each participant must be endorsed by their state nurses association and class size is limited to 24 nurses each year. The program consists of in-person sessions in Washington, DC followed by multiple bi-monthly one-hour conference calls scheduled to accommodate varying time zones and work schedules. Topics include how to conduct a political environmental scan; bill analysis process; coalition building; how to prepare and deliver testimony; and the value of a political action committee (PAC). Each participant is required to collaborate with their state nurses association to choose a policy issue and related legislative actions to focus on during the year. The participant will report to ANA mentors and the state nurses' association about the results of these activities. Naturally, there is a cost associated with this program. Candidates are responsible for transportation, uncovered meals, incidentals, and the $500 registration fee. However, all except one meal is covered in Washington by ANA, and ANA also pays for hotel accommodations. The American Nurses Foundation has some scholarship funds available subject to a match by the individual or state nurses' association (MNORN, 2021).

Another program is the Minnesota Nursing Community Policy Forum where all nursing organizations in the state meet to discuss common policy issues and strategies. Since 2018, the forum has focused on improving the health of the state's citizens. Five nursing organizations support these principles: support access to affordable, high quality health care (including for those in rural areas); address mental health and suicide prevention; ensure access to on-site school health services for all students; focus on gun safety and prevention of gun violence as public health issues; and enable health care workers to practice safely and free from violence (MNORN, 2021).

Every nurse will not be able to attend the previously mentioned programs, but every nurse can gain political awareness and competence. Some will be exposed to political issues and viewpoints in their family, their community, their education program(s), and their organizations. There is no one path to political awareness, but every politically aware individual is curious about their world and is a lifelong learner. This is not just applicable to younger nurses as evidenced in the following quote:

> And to nurse. . . is a field, a road, of which one may safely say: There is no end—no end in what we may be learning every day. There is a well-known Society abroad (for charitable works) of which the Members go through two years' probation on their first entering, but after ten years they return and go through a second probation of one year. This is one of the most striking recognitions I know of the fact that progress is always to be made: that grown-up people, even of middle-age, ought always to have their education going on. But only those *can* learn *after* middle age who have gone on learning up to middle age.
>
> —Nightingale, 2012, pp. 3–4

11

NAVIGATING TODAY'S POLITICAL PROCESS

Politics is a rough and tumble business. It's not for the faint-hearted. I've got bruises and cuts from being in the political arena. But by and large, I understand how to navigate the process.

—Donna Brazile, n.d.

Today's nurses face great opportunities and challenges in navigating the political process, and Donna Brazile's quote is applicable for everyone. After developing political awareness, it will be time to get involved specifically on a local level. No one will ever know everything about each issue and there is a lot of misinformation out there. Nurses must be able to discern fact from fiction. That is beyond the scope of this book, but every nurse navigating today's political process must ask the following questions:

- What is the issue?
- What is the background?
- Where is the evidence?
- Who are the players?
- Who are your allies? Who are your adversaries?
- What is the proposed solution and why?
- What's your position and why?
- What are your options?
- How can you achieve a mutual consensus?

Remember that disagreement will occur in political issues and that the phrase, "because we've always done it this way" must be looked at with suspicion. Navigation takes skill and that needs time and practice. Everyone will stumble at times and make mistakes. That's part of the learning process and the bruises and cuts will heal as you address the challenges in front of you. The political process isn't easy, but it can be rewarding as you grow in legislative advocacy.

Here are comments from other nurses who have successfully navigated these sometimes turbulent, muddy political waters, Michael, Connie, Jo Ann, and Peggy.

1. What has been your involvement in the political process as a nurse?

    a. "There is a blending of policy and politics. Politics is about influencing others to accept your agenda for an issue. This can happen everywhere there are more than two people such as in the office when the group is deciding what to do for the holiday party, in committee meetings, and more formally with regards to electing governmental officials, and the process of creating legislation. Creating policy is done within the matrix of politics. I've only canvassed for one candidate, and he was an ED doc who championed a health care policy that set the stage for the Affordable Care Act. Honestly, I have little interest in supporting elected officials." —Michael
    b. "My involvement in the political process started many years ago when I worked in Maryland. I not only became involved in many professional nursing organizations (which can be considered Political), but also as a member of the Board of the Maryland Nurses Association. I became very involved in the lobbying efforts of the Association. The goals of the lobbying efforts were to impact the health and welfare of the citizens of Maryland, as well as to promote the healthcare workforce agenda. Lobbying with a Nursing or Health Care Association is one way to learn the political process at the front lines of confronting politicians in a meaningful way. More recently I was a consultant to my local state senator in New York State on health care issues that he felt I could be of help in his understanding of those issues. I do continue to attend lobby days at the state level on Nursing and health care issues." —Connie
    c. "I am a Registered Nurse. Except for five years serving as an Army Nurse, my entire career has been in the political arena. My real involvement began as I was about

to graduate from George Washington University with a Master's in Health Administration. I was entering a very slow job market living in Washington, DC and was intrigued by Capitol Hill. I was offered an unpaid internship by the Vietnam Veterans Caucus. This was a newly formed group of young Congressmen who served in various branches of the military during Vietnam and dedicated their legislative efforts to the thousands who had served in our Nation's most unpopular war. They included names like David Bonior, who went on to become House Democratic Whip, Dan Quayle, the former Vice President, and Tom Daschle, the former Senate Majority Leader. I loved attending hearings and meetings, and problem-solving constituent complaints. Like a fly on the wall, I was able to attend important policy discussions and be present when Congress voted on legislation. I migrated to a paying job as a health systems analyst in the Department of Veterans Affairs and was recruited as a volunteer in the 1988 Bush Campaign where I wrote position papers on the graying tsunami of our Nation's veterans. Bush won and I became the first woman to head the National Cemetery Administration of the Department of Veterans Affairs. Of my three Senate confirmed Presidential Appointments, I loved this job the most. I actually had an opportunity to use my nursing skills—problem solving, teamwork, compassion and the ability to exercise calm and control in the face of seemingly insurmountable political and ethical difficulties. Bush lost reelection to Bill Clinton, and I found employment on Capitol Hill; first in the house of Representatives as the staff director of the Veterans Affairs Subcommittee on Health and then later in the Senate as the legislative director for a Republican Senator. I left Capitol Hill to join the newly established Washington office of the American Organization of Nurse Executives, a subsidiary of the American Hospital Association. During my twenty years with what is now the American Organization for Nursing Leadership I have experienced the exhilaration of legislative successes and also bottomless lows and disappointments. Nursing may be the most respected profession but, in my experience, it garners only polite recognition in the Halls of Congress. Nursing has some champions, but no big guns."
—Jo Ann

d. "Early on I became active in our local nursing organization, district 4 of NYSNA, ANA, and NAON. Again, I was pretty verbal about local and state issues related to support of both patients and nurses. Eventually, I became president of that organization, and more active in the state organization. I served on many committees at the state level. The legislative committee was one I served on for many years. Being part of these organizations gave me an opportunity to also meet with state and federal electeds [*sic*] to try to inform them and influence them on nursing and patient care issues. During my career I had also stayed active with our local democratic committee. I also am a member of the NYS Nurse Board. I work with the office of professional discipline to evaluate complaints related to RN and LPN behavior/care. Our primary responsibility is to protect the public. I always try to look at the big picture related to the behavior and the effect on the patient/client. (After retiring) I went into teaching, hopefully influencing the new generation. I encouraged my students to become politically involved by joining a committee at work...either on their own unit or within the hospital. Also encouraged them to join their nursing organization...ANA, NYSNA, or their specialty group." —Peggy

2. How did you become politically aware?

a. "I became interested in politics when Ross Perot ran for president and then only passively. I became aware after becoming a nurse and read the IOM Report on the Future of Nursing and decided that I had a serious knowledge deficit. So, I paid to participate in the defunct Nurse in Washington Internship program which was a powerful experience. Not only did I become informed about how national politics functioned, but how policy and legislation worked. This understanding taught me that real reform takes place at the community level and to a lesser degree at the state level. What I mean by that is implementation of policy occurs at the local level even if the policy is developed at the state level." —Michael

b. "I think I was brought up to be politically aware. My mother was the Chairperson of the Democratic Committee in my hometown in Pennsylvania. As a child I attended many rallies for various candidates and for various issues. I must say it wasn't always fun, but I definitely learned the importance of political engagement if you wanted to make change. I stayed engaged as a member of the student council in high school. The student council was the political body that made decisions impacting student activities and school goals. It was a starting point for me. I remained politically aware through nursing professional organizations, lobbying efforts and indeed running for political office." —Connie

c. "I was born and married into politics. Both my parents were politically involved. My father was a strong union organizer. My mother was a Democratic Committeewoman who shook John f. Kennedy's hand and refused to wash her hand for days. My childhood dentist was my State Senator. In high school I served on the student council. I met my former husband at the White House, and he later became Navy Secretary under Reagan and a U.S. Senator. Over the years, I have had a front row seat into the political landscape from small town politics to the glare of Capitol Hill." —Jo Ann

d. "As a child, my family had political ties. My great uncle was a Republican county supervisor, before the legislator process was developed. A close family friend was chair of the local Democrat Party. As a teenager I got involved in the local Democrat Party, helping out at fundraisers, stuffing envelopes, delivering "propaganda" door to door. When I became an adult, I joined the committee. Although my mom and dad's generation were Republicans, my 3 brothers and I registered Democrat. We were in the John Kennedy era...and had become enthralled with the "what can you do for your country". Although registered Republicans, because that's what most of the community was, my parents were very liberal. They were always involved in events to help out in the community...and the kids followed." —Peggy

3. How do you define legislative advocacy?

   a. "There are several ways to advocate for issues. Most of the legislative policy occurs at the state level and is influenced by groups rather than individuals. An individual trying to talk directly with a state legislator is not easy and it is more likely that any conversation will be with an aide. However, if as a member of an organization, there is a good chance that the legislator will find time to talk—especially one in their first term. As the legislator gains more seniority, the less accessible they are. Advocacy is probably more effective if one is selected to serve on an advisory committee or leads an influential organization such as a state association for defense attorneys or the AARP." —Michael

b. "Legislative advocacy consists of engaging with legislators on the local, state or federal level in an attempt to influence policies and legislation. It is the most direct way for people and teams to make changes in government policies. This includes helping legislators draft a measure for change or helping to introduce legislation that can help to benefit people or organizations. It can also be a way to stop bills that will hurt the public or specific organizations. Advocacy focuses on educating the legislators about a specific issue. I have learned that there are 3 rules of advocacy: be polite, be prepared and be persistent." —Connie

c. "I define legislative advocacy rather broadly. There is formal and informal advocacy. There is grassroots and grass tops. Advocacy occurs one on one and through expenditures of millions of dollars. It occurs through opinion pieces and social media campaigns. The ultimate result is wanted and hopefully needed change for the better." —Jo Ann

4. What have you accomplished from your involvement in the political realm?

    a. "Very little if any. I stopped trying and shifted my focus to supporting activities that empower nurses to get off the sideline and become active in their community organizations as leaders. There they will learn the ropes of politics and policy so that in the future, they can be recognized by legislators and state administrators as valuable contributors to healthcare policy." —Michael

    b. "Over my many years of engaging in the professional and political arena I do feel that my voice has been heard. Some examples include defeating mandatory staffing rations in New York State until 2022. As a nurse leader, I have, as many nurse leaders did as well, advocated to allowing the nursing leadership in the hospitals and nursing homes determine safe staffing and how to accomplish that.

Although there are now mandatory ratios in nursing homes in New York State, each hospital can submit a staffing plan to the State Board of Nursing which will be approved by them. Not truly a mandated staffing ratio. Other legislation that I have lobbied for over the years includes Women's rights to an Abortion; Health Care for All; and Compassionate Care Laws. I was able to be a consultant to my former state senator on health care legislation which I do believe did influence many of his actions." —Connie (Her activity as a candidate will be described in a later chapter.)

c. "Looking back, I can speak to two significant pieces of legislation impacting veterans and numerous changes to appropriations for nursing, additions to the Affordable Care Act, and expansions to nursing practice. None of the changes were accomplished by a single person but through the efforts and continued support of individuals and communities that were committed to a shared goal.

I am so proud of playing a role in the development and passage of PL 104-262, the Veterans Health Care Eligibility Reform Act of 1996. This law completely revamped how the VA delivered care. The legislation moved the VA from a system that delivered episodic disability services into a comprehensive system that enrolled veterans into a comprehensive system of care. This remains the standard for VA healthcare today.

The other legislation of which I am proud to played a role was my decision as the head of the National Cemetery Administration to significantly expand the use of columbarium. This change which was not initially popular, allowed national cemeteries to remain open for burials during the heightened demand for burial space with the passing of the World War II generation. I also championed the installation of cutting-edge technology which digitized century-old paper burial records within the National Cemetery Administration making cemeteries an important resource for researchers and safeguarded American history. For these accomplishments, the National Cemetery Administration was recognized as a beacon of consumer excellence in the provision of government services.

In the nursing arena, the passage of the Nurse Reinvestment Act of 2004 streamlined educational funding and greatly improved upon the administration of the aging Title VIII Nursing Education Programs. Nursing education and practice also were advanced through the input of specific nursing-directed amendments included in the landmark Affordable Care Act." —Jo Ann

d. (Peggy's accomplishments in elected office will be described in a later chapter.)

5. What challenges have you faced?

   a. Before becoming a nurse at age 50, I had no frame of reference to the environment of professionalism and over the course of my journey had to learn how to be a professional. The way that I present myself, the approach I use in difficult conversations was developed by trial and error. I did not have a mentor per se and that gave me an epic disadvantage. But I also think there is an opportunity for nurses to learn how to mentor and mentee. We are pretty good at lecturing and clinical practice but could do better helping one another. My friend convinced me to retry a doctoral program because I was convinced, I was not smart enough. She said, 'I'll be your sherpa' She did, and I did. If she had not, I would not have." —Michael
   b. "There are many challenges when stepping into the political arena. Whether as a health care leader (chief nursing officer or the chair of a health care board) or running for political office, you must face your fears first. It does take courage to stand up to the CEO of a healthcare organization and tell him or her that they are wrong and that you cannot support their conclusion or decision. As the chief nurse, you are there to support the mission and vision of the organization and to advocate for the patients and the staff. At times, that may not fit the CEO's needs. I think I grew stronger as a patient, staff and community advocate by learning that I had a voice and using it.

      The challenges you face as an activist and lobbyist are many as well. You need to be able to state your case quickly and with data (if it is needed) to get heard. Generally, you get very little time with legislators to make your case so use the time wisely. Do your homework and see what the main points are that will sell your case. It is not easy, but you can make a difference." —Connie (Connie's challenges in running for elected office will be described in a later chapter.)

c. "My entire experience in nursing advocacy has been a challenge. Although nursing is respected, it has no real recognizable champions. Florence Nightingale has been dead for over 100 years, and no one has yet to emerge as a voice for the profession. Nursing has no deep pocketed political action committees like technology or pharmaceutical companies. Nursing associations can be tribal in their approach to what is best for the profession." —Jo Ann

d. "There have been many challenges. There are still people who do not think women should hold positions of power... especially when you are in a minority caucus." —Peggy

6. What advice do you have for other nurses who are unsure about how to navigate the political process?

   a. "Become actively engaged! Join your nurses' association as a member of a committee and state board of directors. Attend local and, if possible, state governmental meetings to observe how they function. Join the board of directors for a community organization such as the Boys and Girls Club, Humane Society, or advocacy organization. Find a mentor who is competent and one you would like to emulate. Evaluate yourself based on what skills are needed and what you need to improve and identify your personal hot button for social reform. While you may be a competent nurse, you may not be comfortable at public speaking or adhering to Robert's Rules of Order. Also, sitting on a board requires you to understand financials since there you have fiduciary accountability. Speaking in public, or at board meetings could be improved by joining the local Toastmasters group—not to mention gaining confidence when you hear the sound of your own voice. To become an advocate and reformer, it takes a personal choice. Then, create a personal professional development plan that will support you in this journey to become competent in the environment of advocacy, politics, and reform. I used the nursing process as a guide to create my own plan. Honestly, I have achieved pretty close to nothing as far as I can see except to become prepared to achieve. Maybe someday." —Michael

b. "The best advice I can give to those nurses who are unsure is to take the first step. Join your professional nursing or healthcare organization. See how they are approaching the political arena. Participate in drafting documents for lobbying. That does give you insight as to what the politicians may want from you. Become a leader in your organization or a professional organization so you know what the politics looks like at that level. Offer to be a consultant to your local senator or congressperson. These are ways to test the waters to see where you want to go in your political future. The most important advice is to Listen—not to react but to be open to the political landscape in front of you." —Connie

c. "I have been asked this question many times and my answer is always the same. Find your passion and go for it. Educate yourself on the issues and have a basic understanding of the governmental process. Remember that your elected official is a public servant and serves at the pleasure of his or her constituents, this includes you. Put your toe in the water by joining a group and try volunteering for a person or issue that aligns to your political beliefs. Be willing to accept that most efforts will not move mountains and learn to take pleasure from being part of small but significant changes." —Jo Ann

d. "I always tell nurses who are interested in politics...start with your profession first...then move into the public arena." —Peggy

You've heard from nurses who have navigated the political process. Their approaches and results have varied, but each has wisdom to share with novices beginning their journey in the political realm. To succeed, you must first begin by taking a single step. That may be joining a committee in your organization, a professional nursing association, or a community group that will feed your passion. Find a mentor who will help you gain the knowledge you need to be effective. Develop a team that will collaborate with you to advance the organization, group, or issue. Ask questions and seek advice as you learn the ropes. Listen carefully and realize that nothing is accomplished without perseverance and persistence. Changes may be small or incremental over time, but changes can occur. Most of all, navigating the political process is a team effort. Be sure to practice gratitude in your dealings with your team and the legislators in the process. You can do this!

12

NURSES IN THE POLITICAL ARENA

> *I've had a lot of careers in my life. When I think about it, I think every piece of that—from being a nurse, a farmer, dealing with real estate—has added to a skill set that I would have been able to use throughout my political career.*
>
> —Patty Judge, n.d.

Patty Judge is a registered nurse who served as lieutenant governor of Iowa 2007 to 2011. She also was the first woman to serve Iowa as secretary of agriculture from 1998 to 2006. In 2016, she was the Democratic nominee for U.S. Senate from Iowa, but lost the general election to Sen. Charles Grassley (Ballotpedia).

Once nurses have mastered navigating the political process, the next logical step is running for office locally, statewide, or nationally. Two of the nurses in the last chapter have run for office locally with differing results. There has never been a nurse in the U.S. Senate, but several have served in the House of Representatives in the last 20 years. Currently three nurses are in the House and more are in state and local governments (Summers & Gordon, 2022).

STATE NURSE LEGISLATORS

The last figures for state legislators who are nurses were reported in January 2022. At that time, 76 nurses out of 7,383 state legislators were nurses (0.01%) in 36 states. The breakdown of these nurse legislators is:

- 14 senators;
- 62 representatives;

- 37 Democrats;
- 39 Republicans; and
- 73 of 76 serving on health-related committees.

Current updates since the November 2022 election are not yet available (Curley & Hannan, 2021).

PAST NURSES IN CONGRESS

Here are the stories of the nurses who have served in the U.S. House of Representatives. Their stories and accomplishments may encourage future nurses to seek election to Congress, or even the U.S. Senate.

Rep. Eddie Bernice Johnson (D TX-30) 1993 to 2023

The first RN to be elected to Congress was Eddie Bernice Johnson (D-TX) who was elected in 1992 and served from 1993 to 2023, retiring at the end of the 117th Congress in January 2023. Rep. Johnson grew up in Texas, moved to Indiana after high school to earn a nursing certificate from St. Mary's College at the University of Notre Dame, and returned to Texas where she received a BSN from Texas Christian University and a Master of Public Administration from Southern Methodist University. She became the first Black nurse to become Chief Psychiatric Nurse at the Dallas VA Hospital. The Voting Rights Act of 1965 enabled Blacks to register and vote as well as run for elected office. Johnson began her political rise by running for a seat in the Texas House of Representatives in 1972 and won in a landslide. In 1986 she was elected to the Texas Senate and served there from 1986 until elected as a Democrat to the U.S. Congress representing the 30th District. Rep. Johnson had a distinguished career in Washington, serving as chairperson of the Congressional Black Caucus and became the first Black and first woman to chair the Subcommittee on Water Resources and Environment where she sponsored the Water Resources Act, which was enacted over President Bush's veto. Rep. Johnson introduced the National Nurse Act of 2011, which elevated the importance of the CNO (chief nursing officer) of USPHS (United States Public Health Service) and recognized that nurses can promote social justice and wellness for Americans. She was a strong advocate for science, technology, engineering, and math (STEM) education, and supported grants to increase the number of underrepresented minorities receiving STEM degrees and expanding the number of college faculty members from underrepresented groups (house.gov, 2022).

Rep. Lois Capps (D CA-22, 23, 24) 1998 to 2017

Rep. Lois Capps had an unusual path to Congress. She received a BSN from Pacific Lutheran University, a master's in religion from Yale University, and a master's in education from the University of California Santa Barbara. She worked as a head nurse and nursing instructor at Yale New Haven Hospital and as a staff nurse in Hamden, CT before she and her husband Walter, a theology professor, moved the family to California. There she worked as an elementary school nurse and taught part-time.

After losing in 1994, Walter Capps ran again in 1996 and won a seat in the U.S. House of Representatives. Lois campaigned for him and when he died of a heart attack 9 months into his term, she decided to run for his seat in the special election afterward. She won then and later that year in the general election, beginning her first full term in Congress. Her legislative focus was on nursing, health care, and environmental issues. Rep. Capps served on the Health Subcommittee of the Energy & Commerce Committee and helped pass the Nurse Reinvestment Act of 2002 to address the nursing shortage. She was a consensus builder who crossed party lines to propose bills like the HEART for Women Act; the National Pediatric Research Network Act; the Veteran Emergency Medical Technician Support Act; and the Domestic Violence Survivors Protection Act with bipartisan support. Rep. Capps also led efforts to enact environmental protections, combat global warming, and promote clean energy initiatives. She did not run for reelection in 2016, opting to return home to her family and community (house.gov, 2017).

Carolyn McCarthy (D NY-4) 1997 to 2015

Carolyn McCarthy entered politics from a family tragedy. When her husband and five others were killed and her son seriously injured by a gunman on a commuter train from New York City to Long Island, she became an advocate for gun control. McCarthy graduated from the Glen Cove Nursing School and worked as a nurse in the intensive care unit of Glen Cove Hospital for 30 years. Although a registered Republican, McCarthy wasn't active in politics. While caring for her son, she became politically aware and lobbied Congress to support President Clinton's crime bill, including a ban on assault weapons. When her representative came out against the ban, she decided to challenge him for his House seat. Initially, she tried to run as a Republican, but the Nassau County Republican Chairman discouraged her, and instead the Democratic Party supported her run for this office. Not content to be a one-issue candidate, McCarthy joined the Education and Workforce

Committee where she worked to increase resources for healthy school lunch programs, boost program funding for students with special needs, and helped draft the No Child Left Behind Act. When she was appointed chairperson of the Healthy Families and Communities Subcommittee, Rep. McCarthy promoted reforms to support young people in communities impacted by violence, poverty, and drug abuse. She served on the Financial Service Committee, focusing on helping homeowners avoid foreclosure or bankruptcy. Her emphasis on promoting public service led to the Serve America Act that provided grants for nonprofits, increased educational stipends for volunteers, and expanded the definition of public service. Rep. McCarthy was treated for lung cancer in 2013 and decided not to seek reelection. She left Congress in 2015 and in 2018 had been cancer-free for 5 years (house.gov, 2015).

Ann Marie Buerkle (R NY-25) 2011 to 2013

Ann Marie Buerkle graduated from St. Joseph Hospital School of Nursing in Syracuse and was a trauma nurse at Columbia-Presbyterian Hospital in NYC until her family moved back to Syracuse. She earned a bachelor's degree from Le Moyne College and worked as a nurse educator at St. Joseph Hospital for a time, occasionally substituting as a school nurse. As her political awareness grew, she became involved in local politics and earned a law degree at Syracuse University. Her initial runs for office in the county legislature were unsuccessful, but she was appointed to the city council for a short time. Ann Marie was working for a medical malpractice firm when she was appointed as assistant attorney general. She used her healthcare background to join the Surrogate Decision-making Committee for the NYS Commission on Quality of Care, while counseling victims of domestic abuse and volunteering legal services. A conservative active in the Right to Life movement, she ran for Congress to challenge the incumbent Democratic representative after passage of the Affordable Care Act. Rep. Buerkle won by a small margin and served on three committees: Foreign Affairs, Oversight and Government Reform, and Veterans Affairs, where she chaired the Health Committee. She cosponsored a bill to end federal funding for abortion services and sponsored 17 bills, 3 of which became law. Rep. Buerkle collaborated with the Veterans Affairs Committee Chair to sponsor a military assault prevention bill. Defeated for reelection in 2012, she completed her term and subsequently was appointed by President Obama to the U.S. Consumer Product Safety Commission in 2013 and served as acting chair under President Trump from 2017–2019. She currently serves as Principal at Williams & Jensen, PLLC in Washington, DC (house.gov, 2013).

Renee Ellmers (R NC-2) 2011 to 2017

Renee Ellmers worked as a medical assistant in Michigan to pay for her nursing education and graduated from Oakland University with a BSN. When she and her husband, a surgeon, moved to North Carolina to open a medical practice, Renee became active in the local chamber of commerce and community development. Her community activism evolved into political activism in opposition to the Affordable Care Act (ACA), culminating with running for Congress in the second District in 2010. As a novice in the political arena, she recruited a veteran campaign team who focused on a conservative, small government and cutting taxes and spending. Ellmers defeated two candidates in the primary and a seven-term incumbent in the general election with health care as the major issue. In Congress, Rep. Ellmers sat on three committees: Foreign Affairs, Agriculture, and Small Business. Her major legislation in that term was the Creating Jobs Through Small Business Innovation Act. This authorized renewal of federal initiatives to encourage research and development. However, although the Small Business Committee and the Committee on Science, Space, and Technology reported it favorably, the legislation never went to a final floor vote.

Rep. Ellmers was a hard worker and later chaired the Republican Women's Policy Committee. After reelection, she joined the Energy and Commerce Committee and submitted bills on healthcare issues, including the popular Cancer Patient Protection Act which attracted 123 bipartisan cosponsors. This bill did not receive a committee hearing and would have protected funding for cancer treatment from automatic spending cuts in 2013. Returning to the 114th Congress (2015 to 2017), Rep. Ellmers continued to focus on multiple health issues. Despite her opposition to the ACA, she partnered with a Democratic colleague from North Carolina to help those on Medicare access the latest medical technology.

Redistricting in 2016 moved voters from an adjoining district into her second district, resulting in Ellmer's primary loss. In 2017 she became a regional director of the Department of Health and Human Services and worked as an RN during the COVID-19 Pandemic. In 2019 she launched an unsuccessful campaign for lieutenant governor of North Carolina and for Congress in 2021 (house.gov, 2019).

Diane Black (R TN-6) 2011 to 2019

Diane Black earned an associate degree in nursing from Anne Arundel Community College in Maryland and a BSN from Belmont University in Nashville, Tennessee. She worked as a nurse before seeking elected office and maintained her licensure throughout her political career. After serving in the Tennessee House of Representatives and Senate, Black successfully ran for Congress in 2010 and served from 2011 to 2019. As a freshman legislator, she was appointed to the Ways and Means Committee, which writes the tax laws. Since she had budgetary experience from her years in the state legislature, she also joined the House Budget Committee. In these committees, she supported comprehensive tax reform and worked on healthcare policy. During this time, she introduced the Student and Family Tax Simplification Act to make higher education more affordable through tax credits. She also sponsored a bill to modify requirements to receive Medicaid, which became law in 2011. She also supported the No Budget, No Pay Act that held Members' pay if they did not pass a budget on time, which became law in 2013. In 2017 Rep. Black became the first woman to chair the Budget Committee, where she continued to focus on reducing the national debt and balancing the budget. In 2017 Rep. Black decided to run for governor rather than running for reelection in the House. She lost that primary race and retired from Congress in January 2019 (house.gov, 2020).

CURRENT NURSES IN CONGRESS

As of 2023, there are three registered nurses currently serving in the House of Representatives—Cori Bush, Jen Kiggans, and Lauren Underwood. Here are their stories:

Cori Bush (D MO-1) 2021 to present

Cori Bush received a diploma in nursing from Lutheran School of Nursing in St. Louis, Missouri. She also became a faith leader, community organizer, and ordained pastor. Before studying nursing, Cori worked at a local preschool for minimum wage. She experienced partner abuse, eviction, and two traumatic pregnancies, including a son who required ventilator support after a premature birth. This experience made her an advocate for Black maternal health. She protested as a nurse and clergy member by providing triage care and resources after the murder of Michael Brown in Ferguson, MO. Cori ran unsuccessfully for the

U.S. Senate in 2016 and for the House of Representatives in 2018. She successfully won election in 2021 to the House of Representatives; beginning her term in January 2021, she became the first Black woman and first nurse to represent Missouri in Congress. She was reelected in 2022 and is serving her second term in Congress. Rep. Bush serves on the House Judiciary Committee and the House Oversight Committee. She is a progressive who advocates for police reform, abortion rights, Medicare for All, and supports Black Lives Matter. Rep. Bush has also introduced legislation to end homelessness by 2025 (congress.gov, 2021).

Jen Kiggans (R VA-2) 2023 to present

Jen Kiggans was a naval aviator who served 10 years as a helicopter pilot, including 2 deployments to the Persian Gulf. After leaving the military, she studied nursing at Old Dominion University and Vanderbilt University School of Nursing, becoming an adult geriatric nurse practitioner. She worked in several long-term care facilities and as a primary care provider for a practice in Virginia Beach. Jen first ran for office in 2019 and was elected to the Virginia Senate. In her three sessions there, she successfully championed legislation to establish a military spouse liaison, promote election security, and advocate for patients, families, and caregivers in long-term care settings. Elected in 2022, Rep. Kiggans is beginning her first term in the House of Representatives. She serves on the House Armed Services Committee, the House Committee on Natural Resources, and the House Committee on Veterans Affairs (house.gov, 2023).

Lauren Underwood (D IL-14) 2019 to present

Lauren Underwood earned a BSN from the University of Michigan, where she took a course that stimulated her interest in nursing politics and healthcare policy. She received a MSN/MPH from Johns Hopkins University. After graduating, she began a career at Health and Human Services as a senior advisor and teacher for future nurse practitioners in the Georgetown University's online master's program. Returning to Chicago, Lauren worked at a Medicaid-managed care provider to ensure high-quality, cost-efficient care. When her congressman voted for a healthcare proposal that would have allowed states to weaken coverage for people with pre-existing conditions, Lauren decide to run for Congress. In the beginning, it was a struggle, but she prevailed and began her first term in Congress in January 2019 as the first person of color and the first millennial to represent her community in the House.

She serves on the Committee on Appropriations, and in her first term, Rep. Underwood wrote four bills signed into law by President Trump. She has been reelected twice and her signature legislation is a package of 12 bills called the Momnibus, which is designed to reverse preventable maternal health disparities for Black women. One of the Momnibus bills focused on veterans and was signed into law by President Biden in 2021. Rep. Underwood is co-founder and co-chair of the Black Maternal Health Caucus which advances policy solutions to improve maternal health outcomes and end disparities (house.gov, 2023 & Cramer, 2023).

This is a glimpse into the lives of the registered nurses who previously served and continue to serve in the U.S. Congress. Each story is different, but all reflect nurses who decided to make a difference on the national level. Each has notched significant accomplishments in their career, both within and outside the federal government. Each has used their nursing knowledge and background to benefit their constituents. You will relate to some more than others, but every story is special and a challenge for anyone reading this to raise the bar even further. The future is up to you!

13

NURSES AND LOCAL POLITICS

Local politics is just as important as national—and often easier to influence

—Celeste Ng, 2022

Many of today's nurse legislators started in local politics and some prefer the local political scene to state or national office. Often, the public focuses on major national or regional issues and ignores what is happening close to home. There are reasons why local politics matter, and nurses must pay attention to what is happening around them. This is particularly important if nurses decide to run for office themselves. The decisions of local governmental authorities affect community lives and their deliberations are frequently available to the members of the public for observation and interaction. A good example is the city council where citizens can attend open meetings and offer feedback. Council leaders won't always agree with you on an issue, but they should hear the pros and cons of proposals. Because they want your vote, your voice is important and can make a difference in the outcome.

Here are reasons to get involved in local politics:

- Daily lives are affected by local politics. If you don't bring up issues impacting your community, they may never be addressed;
- Our first line of government is local elected officials. They should be accessible to the average citizen and most want to make the community better. If you don't share your concerns or your vision for the future, your voice won't be heard;

- Participation in local politics is essential to our representative Republic. Together, we can create communities where we can find common ground;
- Your local government's charter provides citizens with the rights to vote and petition, and freedom of speech;
- Local issues and politics often establish precedent for state and national politics;
- It's easier to rally support for local issues;
- Local and state politics determine educational priorities and a good place to begin is with local school board elections;
- Localities have the ability to change laws by petition on state or local ballots;
- Local politicians are easier to hold accountable than national ones;
- Remember to think globally and act locally. Local issues and resulting changes can attract the attention of national media, creating awareness of global issues stemming from these local changes (Deen, 2022).

Now that nurses understand why they must be involved in local politics, the next question is how to do it. The skills discussed in policy, social challenges, advocacy, board service, and gaining political awareness are applicable here. One characteristic nurses have that others don't when running for office is that they are nurses. Nurses' skills are well-suited to public office. Their skills include:

- Listening to understand the problem or issue;
- Expertise in communication with others;
- Effective translation about complex issues into useful results;
- Skillful collaborators and negotiators;
- Effective conflict management; and
- Seeing community issues through a patient's lens to determine a feasible solution (aana.org, 2023).

No one runs for election alone. It takes a village of like-minded advocates to determine what office to select, stake your position(s), plan a campaign, get out the vote, and hopefully win the election. It's important to remember that even an unsuccessful campaign and loss will better prepare you for future elections. Many of our past and current legislators lost the first time, but learned from the experience for a future successful outcome.

ASK QUESTIONS

Many people think they have to know everything before running, which is impossible. It's important to care about the constituency represented, to listen, and to learn. No one learns without asking questions—many of them. If it's a school board or local council, ask people who have run before, election supervisors, people who have served in the role, or even a current member. Ask many questions before you announce your candidacy, including:

- What is the daily responsibility in the position;
- How large of a team is needed;
- How much money must be raised;
- How does campaigning work; and
- Is it a partisan or non-partisan race? (Parks & Weiner, 2019)

DO YOUR RESEARCH

Research helps you decide which voter segment to target and how to do it. If it's your first run for office, you probably can't hire a political consultant and may not have a local political veteran to mentor you in this process. You need to attend community meetings and learn about local issues as well as talk with political and civic influencers about their perspectives. Attending county events with multiple issue-based and public organizations will help clarify your position to persuade local voters. Understanding the concerns of your community will help determine your campaign message. Demographics are important. The local census office or electoral office can give you information about the number of eligible voters who haven't registered yet and the number who are first time and repeat voters. Then, you need to determine the vote goal and the number you need to win (Narayanan, 2022).

FIGURING VOTE GOAL AND WIN NUMBER

To win an election, you need more votes than your competitor. That sounds trite, but it's important to determine the number of votes required to win. The formula for this is simple:

> **Step1**: Project turnout by multiplying the current number of registered voters by the percentage turnout in the last 3 similar elections: 20% × 4,500 = 900

Step 2: Set goal by dividing projected turnout by 2 and adding 1 to get the win number: 900/2 + 1 = 451

Step 3: Determine vote goal by multiplying projected turnout by .52: 900 × .52 = 468

Using this calculation, you project that winning by 52% requires 468 votes (Parks & Weiner, 2019).

RESEARCH FINDINGS

Now that you know the number needed to win, and that an average turnout is 20%, you must target to canvass twice the number of these voters so you can win the majority. No politician focuses on everyone. Limited resources should target voter segments where you can get maximum impact. If running for the school board, it's wise to focus on families with school-age children. Your local election board can give you targeted information on request. For this cost, you will get party registration and addresses of your district's registered voters to help you target your campaign (Parks & Weiner, 2019).

Research on your opponent is vital. How much support does the opposing candidate have? Which voter segment supports them and why? If the majority of your opposition's support is from voters 60 and older, you can focus much of your outreach and messaging on younger voters. This can be an extensive process and requires a few experts to complete this research (Narayanan, 2022).

You need to establish a campaign committee and register it. The campaign committee is a legal business entity, and a campaign checking account is an essential step. Seek advice from someone who is acquainted with the specific laws in your state and never neglect these important steps (Narayanan, 2022).

After your research, you should be able to determine your campaign message, decide your target voter segment, know which office to seek, and establish a campaign plan. The campaign plan is the roadmap from the beginning to election day. It includes the following:

1. **Political environment:** Where do the voters stand? What are your opponent(s) policies and issues?
2. **Demographics and targeting:** How would you target the voters based on gender, age, ethnicity, religion, occupation, and ideology?

3. **Campaign issues and message:** What is your core message? How does it relate to your issues?
4. **Communication plan:** How do you get the message across? How do you get press coverage?
5. **Grassroots outreach:** How do you plan your ground game with volunteers? How do you plan in advance for absentee ballots and election day activities?
6. **Budget:** What is the budget for each task?
7. **Fundraising:** What methods will you use? What are the events and major donors needed to meet fundraising goals?
8. **Timeline:** What are the deadlines for each activity and team?
9. **Staffing:** What are the key roles and important responsibilities for these members? (Narayanan, 2022)

GETTING ON THE BALLOT

Now, you need to get on the ballot. Start with the county elections website or the state's secretary of state office to find deadlines and forms to submit. Getting on a primary ballot varies in different states. In some states, you just complete paperwork, file with the state's election office, and pay any required fees. These filing fees may be waived in some states by obtaining 2% of signatures from district party members. In other states, you must submit a petition with the signatures of a certain number of registered voters from the same party. This number varies by state. Other states conduct party conventions where the party selects candidates for the primary. Unselected candidates may still qualify by submitting a petition. A few states have primaries where every candidate runs on the same ballot after collecting a specific number of signatures and completing required paperwork. States can also choose not to hold primary elections and pick nominees at a convention (democracydocket.com, 2022).

In nonpartisan races, candidates must meet the qualifications and file all required forms. It is essential to meet all deadlines. Independent candidates usually must obtain a larger number of signatures to be on the ballot. If the candidate doesn't win the party's nomination or collect enough signatures to qualify for the ballot, there is one option available—run as a write-in candidate. Besides asking voters to write your name on their ballot, most states require that write-in candidates register with the state prior to the election to be counted, and votes are discarded if the candidate hasn't registered before the election (democracydocket.com, 2022).

ASSEMBLING YOUR ELECTION TEAM

Now, you must build your election team. For a local election, it doesn't have to be large, but members must know the local community and be skilled enough to support you. Naturally, the first place to look is at family and friends to help with campaigning efforts. Delegate tasks that support their strengths based on their experiences and personal skills. Connections with local celebrities or influencers will be beneficial to communication and outreach strategies. Volunteers are essential for headquarters tasks and ground support. Their enthusiasm will help motivate the campaign. Remember, this is not a sprint, and you don't want to wear your volunteers out early in the campaign.

There are four paid roles required in a successful campaign: campaign manager, event or fundraising coordinator, chief volunteer coordinator, and treasurer or finance director. You may also want to invest in some digital technologies so the team has the right tools to handle the workload.

When the team is assembled, you need to determine poster designs, literature text, and design and layout for mailers, yard signs, and brochures. It would be helpful if one of the team members can create designs for campaign materials and forms for volunteers and donors. Meaningful slogans are also powerful campaign assets (Narayanan, 2022).

LOCAL CAMPAIGNING

Begin with a formal announcement that you are running for office in a central location with high traffic and that is patronized by your supporters. Advertise the event so many supporters can attend and invite local press and a respected office holder or community leader who will speak in support of you. This is the first opportunity to get your message out. You'll want to rehearse it a few times, and if needed, review it with the local political party. Your message must be clear and motivating.

Now, it's time to hit the road. In local elections, this means door-to-door canvassing where you meet potential voters face-to-face. Your campaign should have figured out who you need to meet in person, and you need to maintain a voter file to track your communication with each one. All communication with a voter should be updated to personalize and improve your relationship with that person. Other tactics include newspaper ads, billboards, radio ads, TV spot ads, and local magazines. Calculate costs to get the best bang for money spent. Your communication manager can monitor your campaign's Facebook and Twitter accounts, and you can use your own social media to share why you decided to run. Phone text messages are also a powerful communication strategy. Ask supporters to opt-in to SMS (Short Message Service) updates from you and text them about events to encourage participation, identify supporters, and mobilize volunteers (Narayanan, 2022).

FUNDRAISING

Never volunteer to pay for the entire campaign and election costs. Running for office is not cheap, but you don't have to be wealthy. You just have to know how to raise funds to pay expenses. A fundraising plan should be part of the campaign strategy and needs to start early in the process. Check campaign finance laws for the state to ensure compliance with amount raised, individual donations, and how to log donations. Write down your expenses (e.g., website domain, campaign office, stamps, campaign materials) and determine how much you need to raise. Begin by asking friends, family, neighbors, and colleagues as you perfect your approach. You are not asking for yourself. The money is to support change that you and the donor believe in and you can't be afraid to ask. You have to believe in yourself and what you can accomplish. This makes asking easier. If you are representing a political party, members will also seek funding for you. Financial support from community leaders will give your campaign credibility. Fundraising can also occur at your sponsored events. Remember that the amount you raise at these events must cover the organizing costs and overhead for the event with funds left over for the campaign. Your goal is a steady flow of funds from supporters and large single donations from your political champions. When done correctly, fundraising should also be good marketing for the campaign (Narayanan, 2022; Parks & Weiner, 2019).

GETTING OUT THE VOTE

The final step is getting out the vote. You can remind voters in your contacts that voting is essential for change to occur. You may also have a few voters who need rides to the polls and volunteers can be sure they get there. Now, you wait for the (hopefully positive) results.

REAL STORIES

Let's hear from your nurse colleagues who have run for elected office locally.

Connie's story

"Post retirement I became very involved in my county's Democratic Committee, and as a member learned even more about the process and how to shape the candidates' views to meet the needs of our community. This is how I became a candidate for a county board position. I was selected by my Democratic Committee to run for the county Board of Directors to represent my district. It was felt that, in the time of the COVID-19 outbreak, a healthcare professional, especially a nurse, could bring the messages forward to the county government that were needed to shape the plans going forward. I was also recognized for my engagement as chair of a nursing home board and chair of a hospice board. My supporters felt that these were areas that our county was not strongly supportive of and that a change in attitude was necessary for the well-being of the county. Living in a very rural county in Upstate New York also allowed me to know of many other issues facing our rural economy, including the impact of poor Broadband capability. Again, I could speak to the need for this as we expanded in the direction of virtual healthcare platforms. My campaign slogan was Otsego Strong—the county name and the recognition that we needed to do more to keep our county moving forward. I did not win the seat, but I have influenced my opponent in that race. He now attends all town meetings which he did not before. I feel that I made him feel that he needed to be more accountable to his constituents and he is."

Peggy's Story

"Ten years ago, our county legislator moved to another position. He reached out to me to run for his seat. I resisted, but continued to be encouraged by others. So, I jumped in...not planning to get elected, but I did...five times. As a legislator, I oversee staffing in the health department. I advocate for positions and pay and benefits. Even though the county has no direct responsibility on nursing homes, I actively engage with our state delegation and the NYS Department of Health to advocate for care of the patients. Recently, I have been displaced as chair of health and human services because I will not be silenced about unfair behavior and issues that affect the most disadvantaged in our community. This will be my last year as an elected legislator. 10 years is enough. I must say that I do believe people supported and liked me because I am a nurse. I think I am transparent and trustworthy. I hope that is a reputation nurses continue to have. One of my favorite times was working side by side with nurses in our health department administering vaccinations. It gave me an opportunity to know the staff and interact with the public—always my favorite things. Just another little note...last campaign my opponent spent $88,000 trying to beat me. I spent about $10. I won by 12 points."

ADVICE FOR FUTURE NURSE CANDIDATES

> As a political candidate, know what the main concerns of your constituents are. In the political world running for an office as a novice can be difficult. Create your campaign around the major issues you are learning from your constituents. Hold round tables and open forums to meet the people that you will be serving. Develop a campaign committee as it is impossible to do this alone. Be prepared for people judging you and calling you out on issues that they do not agree with. That was the biggest challenge I felt. The most important advice is to listen—not to react, but to be open to the political landscape in front of you.
>
> —Connie

> I always tell nurses who are interested in politics. . . start with your profession first. . . then move into the public arena.
>
> —Peggy

Are you interested in running for an elected office after reading this chapter? How will you make a difference in the future?

14

THE FUTURE OF NURSES IN POLICY AND POLITICS

The most effective way to influence your future in nursing is to be involved in politics.

—Dr. Jayesh Patidar, 2013

Not all nurses will run for elected offices, but all nurses need to be knowledgeable about issues impacting their profession, their patients, their communities, their families, and themselves. Speaking out can take many forms—researching legislators' positions, casting an informed vote in elections, writing letters to the editor of local newspapers, volunteering for civic groups (e.g., PTA, library, senior centers), donating to local causes (e.g., food banks, Boys & Girls Clubs), and serving on local boards (e.g., neighborhood associations, nonprofits addressing hunger, homelessness). It's important to find something that ignites your passion because that will determine your level of involvement and enjoyment in advocacy for causes and policies to improve your community and the lives of your fellow citizens. Many of the chapters here will help guide you in your future activities and growth as you focus on social challenges and your ability to make a positive difference.

Some professional organizations help interested individuals learn the fundamentals of the political process and how to run for office as well as providing resource support. The tips in the preceding chapter reflect these organizations. Although nursing specialty organizations and state nurses' associations conduct education programs, such as the American Nurses Advocacy Institute, to help nurses gain political competence and develop advocacy skills, no single nursing program has taught nurses the nuts and bolts of running for (and actually) winning an elected office (MNORN, 2021). That is about to change.

The future will require nurses to expand their skills in the political arena, and some will accept the challenge to seek political office. Unfortunately, advocacy skills are different from those required for political engagement at the candidate level. Although most nurses are positive about advocacy (whether or not they participate in it), some nurses have a negative perception of politics based on their own biases and perceptions. Before a nurse can consider running, he or she must decide that the political journey is worth the effort. No one should seek elected office without believing that their election will make some aspect of the community and the Republic better.

HEALING POLITICS—THE BEGINNING

Current campaign schools vary from one day to a week and even one day a month for 6 months. They also have not specifically targeted nurses until now. Lisa Summers' history reflects that of nurses met in earlier chapters. She was engaged in advocacy as a midwife in a state where midwives were few in number and subsequently was a grassroots volunteer in national campaigns in another state. In 2018, Lisa became a faculty advisor to two nurses enrolled in the DNP program at Yale University School of Nursing. One student had run for a state house seat unsuccessfully and the other (Kimberly Gordon) was actively engaged in politics, campaign work, and advocacy at the state and federal level. After discussion with Lisa, they decided to select a DNP project about why nurses are underrepresented in elective offices. Lisa involved members of the Political Science Department at Yale who were interested in electing women to office, but had not considered nurses (Summers, 2023).

As the project evolved, evidence from literature showed that getting similar people (in this case, nurses) together was beneficial to success. Nurses also tend to talk with each other about issues, but don't communicate outside their own circle. Gradually, the idea of a campaign school specific to nurses began to grow, and Lisa and Kimberly decided to develop a program to prepare nurses and midwives with resources and skills to successfully win elections. A program was developed in May 2020, but COVID-19 delayed its start. Because our current political climate is divisive and polarized, they wanted their program to begin the healing process in politics. With this in mind, they created Healing

Politics as a nonpartisan campaign school for nurses to help nurses and midwives share their skills and unique perspectives in political roles that will bring people together and result in better health for everyone. It became a 501©3 nonprofit organization in 2021 (Summers, 2023).

This nonprofit aspect makes Healing Politics a unique campaign school because most provide ongoing political support to participants based on a political party or political inclinations. Nonprofit 501©3 organizations cannot support candidates running for office as individuals, and participants must seek such support after matriculating from political parties or other organizations (e.g., mental health, climate change, political action committees). The organization's mission, vision, and values also delineate it from other campaign schools.

> **Mission:** "Healing Politics is on a mission to inspire, motivate, recruit, and train nurses and midwives to run for elected office up and down the ballot while building a culture of civic engagement within the professions" (Healing-Politics.org, 2023).
>
> **Vision:** "We envision a country where every citizen is governed by public policy that is developed by and reflective of the community they live in, where nurses and midwives are actively engaged in the creation of policy that improves the health of the nation" (Healing-Politics.org, 2023).
>
> **Values:**
>
> "We value diversity and strive for equity;
>
> "We value science, basing our work on existing and emerging evidence;
>
> "We value strategic partnerships that will inform our work and strengthen our impact;
>
> "We value innovation in developing solutions to barriers, real and imagined; and
>
> "We value empowerment, recognizing and celebrating the potential of nurses and midwives" (Healing-Politics.org, 2023).

Healing Politics Inaugural Campaign School for Nurses & Midwives in 2023 will be open to 50 nurses representing political, racial, geographic, socioeconomic, and cultural diversity; providing time for engagement, networking, role-play, and learning in a fast-paced, interactive environment that resembles life on the campaign trail. The 3.5-day program will function as a simulation lab for political nurse novices, including how to present yourself as a nurse and how to leverage that when fundraising. Participants will be asked to raise $200 within 30 days of completing the program in addition to the tuition to sustain the campaign school and practice fundraising skills (Healing-Politics.org, 2023 & Summers, 2023).

A virtual preparatory session titled "Before You Take the Leap: 10 Questions You Must Answer Before Running" will occur prior to the live program so participants can make the most of the experience. Realizing that nurses are well qualified for elective office, Healing Politics is designed to:

- Inspire nurses to run for elected office at all levels of the ballot;
- Identify nurse candidates and develop a community of nurses to support them;
- Provide nonpartisan training to help nurses run and win;
- Promote a nursing culture where colleagues who run are supported; and
- Partner with researchers to expand our knowledge about nurses and midwives in elected office (Healing-Politics.org, 2023).

Sessions will include:

- Welcome or networking reception—an opportunity to interact with multiple people as a candidate would in an actual campaign function;
- How to prepare for a successful campaign by addressing planning, structure, and budget;
- Running an ethical campaign;
- How to operationalize a successful campaign by developing an effective message;
- How to communicate your message to voters and the media;
- How to do fundraising; and
- How to find and track voters as well as getting out the vote on election day (Healing-Politics.org, 2023).

The school's diverse faculty includes three RNs, two of whom serve as state senators and one who is currently a lieutenant governor of another state, two political consultants, one political attorney, and one political media strategist. All will share their extensive knowledge and expertise with participants (Healing-Politics.org, 2023).

One month after the campaign school, a virtual follow-up session will address any questions related to any aspect of the training provided. Because Healing Politics cannot engage in campaign activities for any candidate, this session is an opportunity to clarify any information and its potential applicability in future campaigns. It will also provide an opportunity for graduates to interact and support each other (Healing-Politics.org, 2023).

Although every nurse will not consider a run for elected office, every nurse must be politically aware and willing to support his or her colleagues who decide to take the plunge into electoral politics. The Healing Politics Campaign School is distinctive because it provides resources for mailing list members who are not ready to run but are either interested for the future or only interested in supporting other nurses or midwives. These resources include newsletters, links to nursing media sites, and books about experiences in elected office (Healing-Politics.org, 2023).

As mentioned earlier, nurses are the most trusted profession and have been for the past 21 years (Advisory Board, 2023 & aana.org, 2023). However, the public doesn't really understand what nurses do beyond caring. As Lisa Summers shared, the public needs to know how we leverage technology to keep patients alive and the technical skills we employ in our daily activities. We need to build on that trust so people will understand who we are and what we do. "We need to leverage it at the ballot box" (Summers, 2023).

We have an opportunity as nurses to determine our future and that of our fellow citizens. Whether you run for office or choose to support your colleagues in their races, every nurse has a role to play in that future, starting today!

AFTERWORD

How will we navigate politics in our personal and professional lives?

- Be informed about
    - õ U.S. history from the beginning to today;
    - õ social and policy challenges;
    - õ politics and healthcare.
- Be prepared for
    - õ advocacy;
    - õ political awareness;
    - õ navigating the political process.
- Be involved by
    - õ being an informed voter;
    - õ serving in local organizations or boards;
    - õ advocating for change;
    - õ supporting nurses who run for elected office;
    - õ or running yourself!

Only you can answer this question: Nursing and health care, where is nursing?

ACKNOWLEDGMENTS

This book would not have been possible without the contributions of nurse colleagues who were willing to share their experiences in advocacy, policy initiatives, board service, and politics to inform my readers and myself about how to successfully navigate the policy and the political environment now and in the future.

My sincere thanks to the nurses I interviewed for this book:

- Elizabeth (Liz) Dietz, EdD, RN, CS-NP
- Elizabeth Eugenio Fildes, EdD, RN, CNE, PHNA-BC, FIAAN, FAAN
- Gayle Peterson, RN-BC
- Lisa Summers, DrPH, MSN, RN

and to those who were kind enough to provide their invaluable input:

- Sarah Beckman, MSN, RN
- Peggy Chase, EdD, RN
- Karen Graybeal, MS, RN-BC
- Flora B. Haus, MSN, RN-BC Gerontology
- Connie Jastremski, RN, MS, MBA, ANP
- Michael Polacek, DNP, RN, PMH-BC
- Rachel Ramsey, MSN, RN
- Jo Ann Webb, RN, MHA, FAAN

APPENDIX

POLITICAL PROCESS SURVEY

Hello!

I am currently writing my sixth book for publication titled: *The Politics of Healthcare: Where is Nursing?* and would appreciate your input and advice for nurses about policy and politics.

I am available for any questions. Would you kindly respond to the questions below?

1. What has been your involvement in the political process as a nurse?
2. How did you become politically aware?
3. How do you define legislative advocacy?
4. What have you accomplished from your involvement in the political realm?
5. What challenges have you faced?
6. What advice do you have for other nurses who are unsure about how to navigate the political process?

Thank you!

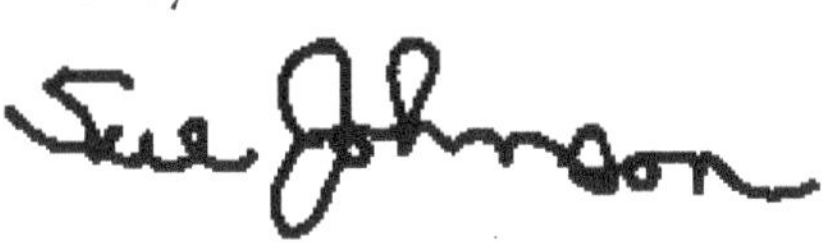

Sue Johnson, PhD, RN, NPD-BC, NE-BC, FAAN
SueJohn126@comcast.net
Cell: XXX-XXX-XXXX

BOARD SERVICE SURVEY

Hello!

I am currently writing my sixth book for publication titled: *The Politics of Healthcare: Where is Nursing?* and would appreciate your input and advice for nurses about board service.

I am available for any questions. Would you kindly respond to the questions below?

1. What preparation (if any) did you have before joining your first board?
2. Did you have a mentor for board service?
3. How do you evaluate board opportunities?
4. What skills do you bring to a board?
5. What have you learned from board service?
6. What advice do you have for nurses seeking board service?

Thank you!

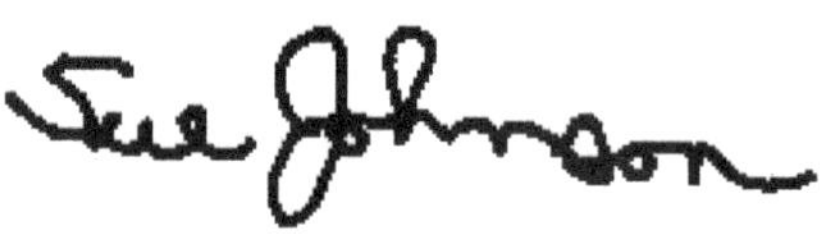

Sue Johnson, PhD, RN, NPD-BC, NE-BC, FAAN
SueJohn126@comcast.net
Cell: XXX-XXX-XXXX

REFERENCES

American Association of Nurse Anesthesiology. (2023). *You Already Possess the Skills Required of Elected Officials.* Retrieved from https://nurseanesthesiology.aana.com/you-already-possess-the-skills-required-of-elected-officials

Advisory Board. (2023, January 18). *Charted: The most trusted professions in America according to Gallup.* Retrieved from https://www.advisory.com/daily-briefing/2023/01/18/trusted-professionals

Alchin, L. (2015, June). *Timeline U.S. Political Parties.* Retrieved from https://www.government-and-constitution.org/history-us-political-parties/timeline-us-political-parties.htm

American Medical Association. (1930). *Sheppard-Towner Act.* Retrieved from https://www.chegg.com/flashcards/quiz-2-17af2854-e832-47ae-9305-53bf458a7840/deck

American Nurses Association. (2010). *Nursing's Social Policy Statement: The Essence of the Profession.* Silver Spring, MD: American Nurses Association.

American Nurses Association. (2015). *Code of Ethics for Nurse with Interpretive Statements.* Silver Spring, MD: American Nurses Association.

American Nurses Association. (2021). *Nursing Scope and Standards of Practice.* (4th, Ed.) Silver Spring, MD: American Nurses Association.

American Nurses Association. (2022). *ANA Political Action Committee.* Retrieved from https://ana.aristotle.com/SitePages/anapac.aspx

American Nurses Association. (2023). *Nursing Priorities.* Retrieved from https://nursesvote.org/issues/

American Nurses Association. (2023, March). Nurses ranked most most honest and ethical professionals for 21st year. *American Nurse Journal, 18*(3), 31. Retrieved from ANA Enterprise News.

American Public Health Association. (2018). *Creating the Healthiest Nation: Advancing Health Equity.* Retrieved from https://www.apha.org/-/media/Files/PDF/factsheets/Advancing_Health_Equity.ashx

National Archives. (n.d.). *America's Founding Documents: The Bill of Rights.* Retrieved from https://www.archives.gov/founding-docs/bill-of-rights

Aristotle. (2000). *Politics.* (B. Jowett, Trans.) Mineola, New York: Dover Publications, Inc.

Ballotpedia. (n.d.). *Patty Judge.* Retrieved from https://ballotpedia.org/Patty_Judge

Bell, J. L. (2017, March 27). *How Dr. McHenry Operated on His Anecdote.* Retrieved from https://boston1775.blogspot.com/2017/03/how-dr-mchenry-operated-on-his-anecdote.html

Block, I. (1969). *Neighbor to the Worlos: The story of Lillian Wald.* New York, NY: Thomas Y. Crowell Company.

boardsource.org. (2020). *The Board's Role in Advocacy.* Retrieved from https://standforyourmission.org/advocacy-your-board/

Brazile, D. (n.d.). *Politics.* Retrieved from http://www.picturequotes.com/politics-is-a-rough-and-tumble-business-its-not-for-the-faint-hearted-ive-got-bruises-and-cuts-from-quote-975403

Breckinridge, M. (1952). *Wide neighborhoods: A story of the Frontier Nursing Service.* Louisville, KY: The University Press of Kentucky.

Cato Institute. (2013). *The Declaration of Independence and the Constitution of the United States of America.* Cato Institute. Retrieved from https://www.cato.org/books/cato-pocket-constitution

Centers for Disease Control. (2015). *Definition of Policy.* Retrieved from https://www.cdc.gov/policy/opaph/process/definition.html

congress.gov. (2021). *Cori Bush.* Retrieved from https://www.congress.gov/member/cori-bush/B001224?q=%7B

Content Team. (2019, January 19). *Public Policy.* Retrieved from https://legaldictionary.net/public-policy/

Cramer, R. (2023). *A life in Congress: Lauren Underwood learns what it means.* Washington Post. https://www.washingtonpost.com/nation/2023/03/04/congresswoman-lauren-underwood-profile/

Curley, D., & Hannan, J. (2021). *Statue Report: State Nurse Legislators 2020–2022.* Retrieved from https://www.nursingworld.org/~4a6c69/globalassets/practiceandpolicy/advocacy/state/9.12.22-status-report--nurse-state-legislators-2020-22.pdf

Deen, L. (2022). *Ten Reasons Why We Should Pay Attention to Local Politics.* US Represented. https://usrepresented.com/2022/09/01/ten-reasons-pay-attention-local-politics/

Democracy Docket. (2022, May 13). *How to qualify for the ballot.* Retrieved from https://www.democracydocket.com/analysis/how-to-qualify-for-the-ballot/

Dietz, L. (2023, February 23). Liz & Sue. (S. Johnson, Interviewer)

Dock, L. (1900). What we may expect from the law. *American Journal of Nursing, 1*(1), 8–12.

Dole, E. (n .d.). *Elizabeth Dole.* Retrieved from https://www.azquotes.com/quote/700782

Donahue, M. P. (2010). *Nursing, the finest art: an illustrated history* (3rd ed.). Maryland Heights, MO: Mosby.

Fildes, E. (2023, February 9). Elizabeth & Sue. (S. Johnson, Interviewer)

Handlin, O. (Ed.). (1966). *The Popular Sources of Political Authority: Documents on the Massachusetts Constitution of 1780.* Belknap Press of Harvard University Press. Retrieved from https://press-pubs.uchicago.edu/founders/documents/bill_of_rightss6.html

Healing-Politics.org. (2023). *Welcome to Healing Politics.* Retrieved from https://healing-politics.org/

Hill, M., & Varone, F. (2021). *The Public Policy Process* (8th ed.). New York, NY. Routledge.

Internal Revenue Service. (2022, June). *Lobbying.* Retrieved from https://www.irs.gov/charities-non-profits/lobbying

Johnson Lewis, J. (2019, November 15). *The Sheppard-Towner Act of 1921.* Retrieved from https://www.thoughtco.com/sheppard-towner-act-of-1921-3529478

Judd, D., Sitzman, K., & Davis, G. (2010). *A history of American nursing: Trends and eras.* Sudbury, MA: Jones and Bartlett Publishers.

Madison, J. (2010). *The Federalist Papers No. 10.* Tribeca Books. Retrieved from http://www.foundingfather.info/federalistpapers/fed10.htms

McCullough, D. (2001). *John Adams.* New York, NY: Simon & Schuster.

Minnesota Organization of Registered Nurses. (2021). *The American Nurses Advocacy Institute.* Retrieved from https://www.mnorn.org/

Narayanan, L. (2022). *A first-time candidate's guide to win local political campaigns.* Retrieved from https://callhub.io/run-local-political-campaign/

National Conference of State Legislatures. (2022, July 11). *Straight Ticket Voting.* Retrieved from https://www.ncsl.org/research/elections-and-campaigns/straight-ticket-voting.aspx

Ng, C. (2022). *Celeste Ng.* Retrieved from https://www.celesteng.com/about

Nurses on Board Coalition. (2022). *Nurses on Boards Coalition.* Retrieved from https://www.nursesonboardscoalition.org/

The Open University. (2019, March 10). *What is politics?* Retrieved from https://www.open.edu/openlearn/society-politics-law/what-politics/content-section-0?active-tab=description-tab

Parks, M., & Weiner, C. (2019). *How to run for office.* Retrieved from https://www.npr.org/2019/10/15/770332855/how-to-run-for-office

Patidar, J. (2013). *Nurses in Politics.* Retrieved from https://www.slideshare.net/drjayeshpatidar/nurses-in-politics

Peterson, G. (2023, February 17). Gayle & Sue. (S. Johnson, Interviewer)

Phaneuf, M., & Donabedian, A. (1976). *The Nursing Audit: Self-Regulation in Nursing Practice* (2nd ed.). New York, NY: Appleton-Century-Crofts.

Postell, D. (2007). *Securing Liberty: The Purpose and Importance of the Bill of Rights.* The Heritage Foundation. Retrieved from https://www.heritage.org/the-constitution/report/securing-liberty-the-purpose-and-importance-the-bill-rights

Price, B. (1932, July). "Politics at Random". *Associated Press Washington Bureau.* Associated Press.

Rose, M. (2018, February 24). *What is Politics*? OurPolitics.net. Retrieved from https://ourpolitics.net/what-is-politics/

Rudolph, L., Caplan, J., Ben-Moshe, K., & Dillon, L. (2013). *Health in All Policies: A Guide for State and Local Govenrments.* American Public Health Association and Public Health Institute, Washington, DC and Oakland, CA.

Summers, L. (2023, March 22). Lisa & Sue. (S. Johnson, Interviewer)

Summers, L., & Gordon, K. (2022, October). Is there a nurse in the House? Or the Senate? *American Nurse Journal, 17*(10), 48.

Szulecki, D. (2023, January). The Top Social Justice Stories of 2022. (D. Szulecki, Ed.) *American Journal of Nursing, 123*(1), 14-15.

Teresa, M. (n.d.). *Mother Teresa Quotes.* Retrieved from https://www.azquotes.com/author/14530-Mother_Teresa

University of Minnesota. (2016). *American Government and Politics in the Information Age* (adapted ed.). Minneapolis, MN: University of Minnesota Libraries Publishing.

University of St. Augustine. (2021, September). *60 Key Nursing Statistics and Trends for 2021.* Retrieved from https://www.usa.edu/blog/nursing-statistics/

United States House of Representatives. (2013). *Buerkle, Ann Marie.* Retrieved from https://history.house.gov/People/Detail/10441

United States House of Representatives. (2015). *McCarthy, Carolyn.* Retrieved from https://history.house.gov/People/Detail/17705

United States House of Representatives. (2017). *Capps, Lois.* Retrieved from https://history.house.gov/People/Detail/11744

United States House of Representatives. (2019). *Ellmers, Renee.* Retrieved from https://history.house.gov/People/Listing/E/ELLMERS,-Renee-(E000291)/

United States House of Representatives. (2020). *Black, Diane.* Retrieved from https://history.house.gov/People/Listing/B/BLACK,-Diane-(B001273)/

United States House of Representatives. (2022). *Johnson, Eddie Bernice.* Retrieved from https://history.house.gov/People/Listing/J/JOHNSON,-Eddie-Bernice-(J000126)/

United States House of Representatives. (2023). *Jen Kiggans.* Retrieved from https://kiggans.house.gov/

United States House of Representatives. (2023). *Lauren Underwood.* Retrieved from https://underwood.house.gov/

Washington, G. (1796, September 19). Washington's Farewell Address Retrieved October 29, 2023, from https://www.senate.gov/artandhistory/history/resources/pdf/Washingtons_Farewell_Address.pdf

Wilkie , K., & Moseley, E. (1969). *Frontier nurse: Mary Breckinridge.* New York, NY: Julian Messner.

Williams, B. (1948). *Lillian Wald: Angel of Henry Street.* New York, NY: Julian Messner.

Zhu, P. (2016). Digitizing boardroom. Pennsauken Township, NJ: BookBaby.

INDEX

www.ingramcontent.com/pod-product-compliance
Lightning Source LLC
LaVergne TN
LVHW101504200926
848483LV00001B/219
* 9 7 8 1 8 0 4 4 1 5 2 7 6 *